MORE THAN 150 HEALTHY AND DELICIOUS RECIPES

you are what you eat™ COOKBOOK

Gillian McKeith, PhD

A PLUME BOOK

PLUME
Published by the Penguin Group
Penguin Group (USA) Inc., 375 Hudson Street, New York, New York 10014, U.S.A.
Penguin Group (Canada), 90 Eglinton Avenue East, Suite 700, Toronto, Ontario, Canada M4P 2Y3 (a division of Pearson Penguin Canada Inc.)
Penguin Books Ltd., 80 Strand, London WC2R 0RL, England
Penguin Ireland, 25 St. Stephen's Green, Dublin 2, Ireland (a division of Penguin Books Ltd.)
Penguin Group (Australia), 250 Camberwell Road, Camberwell, Victoria 3124, Australia (a division of Pearson Australia Group Pty. Ltd.)
Penguin Books India Pvt. Ltd., 11 Community Centre, Panchsheel Park, New Delhi – 110 017, India
Penguin Group (NZ), 67 Apollo Drive, Rosedale, North Shore 0632, New Zealand
(a division of Pearson New Zealand Ltd.)
Penguin Books (South Africa) (Pty.) Ltd., 24 Sturdee Avenue, Rosebank, Johannesburg 2196, South Africa

Penguin Books Ltd., Registered Offices: 80 Strand, London WC2R 0RL, England

Published by Plume, a member of Penguin Group (USA) Inc. Originally published in the UK by Michael Joseph, an imprint of the Penguin Group.

First Plume Printing, January 2011
10 9 8 7 6 5 4 3 2

Ⓟ REGISTERED TRADEMARK — MARCA REGISTRADA

LIBRARY OF CONGRESS CATALOGING-IN-PUBLICATION DATA

McKeith, Gillian.
    You are what you eat cookbook : more than 150 healthy and delicious recipes / Gillian McKeith.
        p. cm.
    "A plume book."
    Companion book to: McKeith, Gillian. You are what you eat: the plan that will change your life. London : Michael Joseph, c2004.
    ISBN 978-0-452-29704-3
    1. Cooking. 2. Vegetarian cooking. 3. Cookbooks. I. McKeith, Gillian. You are what you eat. II. Title.
    TX714.M3839 2011
    641.5'636 — dc22
                                                                                2010041771

Printed in the United States of America

PUBLISHER'S NOTE
The recipes contained in this book are to be followed exactly as written. The Publisher is not responsible for your specific health or allergy
needs that may require medical supervision. The Publisher is not responsible for any adverse reactions to the recipes contained in this book.

Every effort has been made to ensure that the information contained in this book is complete and accurate. However, neither the publisher nor the
author is engaged in rendering professional advice or services to the individual reader. The ideas, procedures, and suggestions contained in this book
are not intended as a substitute for consulting with your physician. All matters regarding your health require medical supervision. Neither the
author nor the publisher shall be liable or responsible for any loss or damage allegedly arising from any information or suggestion in this book.

CONTENTS

MY STORY

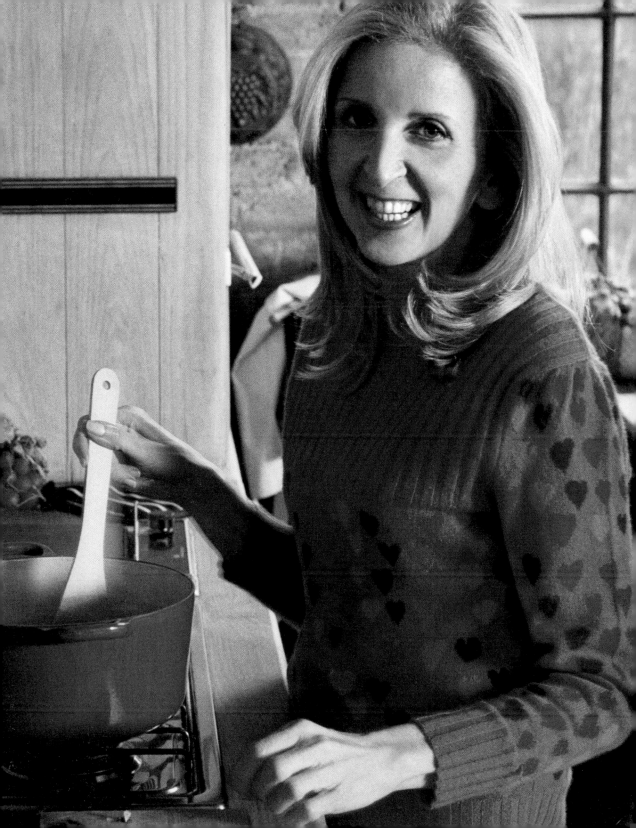

I truly believe anyone can be a great cook as long as they have the will to do it. When I was a wee lass at Perth High School I remember making cheese flan in Home Economics. The funny thing was, I hadn't even tasted the flan because at the time I detested the idea of eating cheese. But somehow I had been so passionate about my recipe that my cooking teacher gave me top marks, because my heart and mind had been in the right place.

My younger brother David had different views about my culinary skills, however, and when we were growing up he spent the entire time complaining to Mom and Dad that I couldn't even toast bread properly. OK, it's true that for some reason my toast always came out pitch-black like coal ... Anyway, David always used to say that I'd burn the house down one day—a statement I took to be completely ludicrous ... until that fateful rainy day when I was 17 and had just received my letter of acceptance into Edinburgh University. I was feeling really excited and preoccupied (as you get with such things)—and, of course, the bread was toasting away in the toaster—when, all of a sudden, the smell of burning wheat seemed to be permeating my bedroom.

I quickly darted into the kitchen, to be greeted by what looked like a scene from *The Towering Inferno*. My toast had caught on fire and the flames had spread to the countertops and walls. I was terrified—not just at the thought of burning down our family home, but at what my dad would say. Then, right on cue, David burst on the scene and quickly and efficiently proceeded to extinguish the fire with buckets of water and heavy wet towels.

So I am no Michelin-star chef—I am just a mother who wants the best for her family, and a holistic nutritionist who wants the best health and purest food for you. I just happen to have developed lots of healthy, fun, and easy recipes over the years as part of my job. The bottom line is that it makes no difference whether you're a Cordon Bleu protégé or a toast-burning pyromaniac: my recipes are quick to prepare—many only take a few minutes—and they're dead simple. If I can make them, anyone can!

Writing these recipes for you and making them readily available was something that was very important to me, because I understand first-hand how essential support like this can be to achieve wellness and a fit body. When I was twenty-something, I lived in Spain and survived on a diet of Spanish éclairs, paella, chocolate, and sangrias. When I got back to Britain I was chubby, had spots all over my face, and felt constantly tired, listless, and unmotivated. A special diet could be my answer, I thought. A simple food plan. So for eight weeks I ate almost nothing but pork deli meats—or, to be precise, three slices of thin ham on two pieces of white bread. And I ate that for breakfast, lunch, and dinner every day. As you can imagine, I felt and looked terrible. Over time, my unhealthy eating habits continued to wreak havoc with my body, energy levels, and general well-being. It was this degeneration in my health that was the key motivating factor in my embarking on a new healthy lifestyle, and a diet of living foods.

When I finally turned my life and health around through natural nutrition and good food, I realized that (a) healthy recipes can be easy to prepare; (b) healthy meals can be quick, exciting, and fun; (c) you can make food taste great even without any experience or training; and (d) healthy food can make you feel and look well, because *you really are what you eat.* All you need is the desire and the will to feel and be well.

The recipes in this book are easy, colorful, and utterly delicious, and I really hope you love them as much as I do. But they're really just the beginning. Once you've gotten a handle on them, I'd like you to feel empowered to experiment, using them as a basis for creating other tasty dishes of your own. All my recipes have the ability to enhance your health and well-being for a far happier, healthier, energized, fitter, and sexier you. And best of all, they won't ever make you fat, which means you can eat as much as you like with them. So it's time to get cooking to your heart's (and tummy's) content.

Wishing you Love and Light, *Gillian*

CHAPTER 1 FOOD PHILOSOPHY

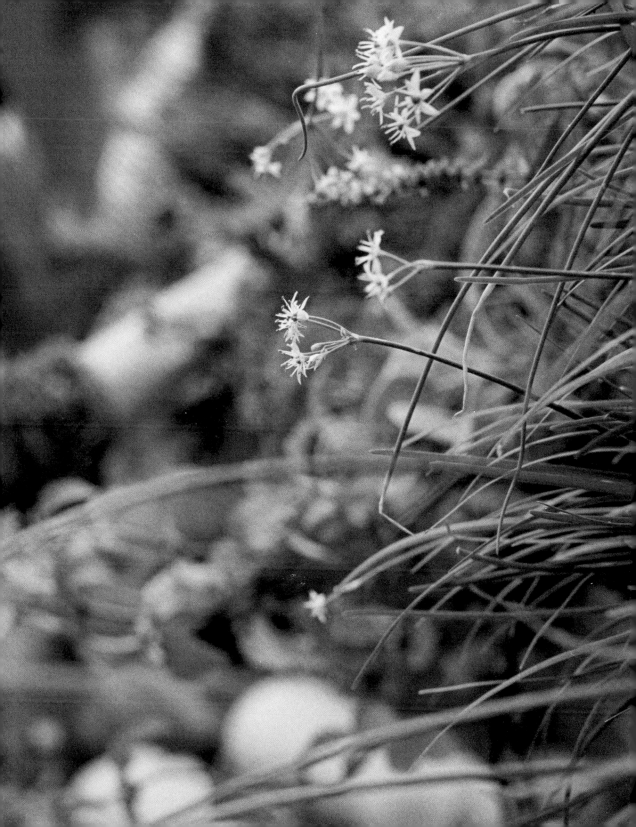

KEEP IT SIMPLE

My food philosophy consists of a few simple guidelines. These are covered in much more detail in the book *You Are What You Eat*. Follow them and you'll be happier, healthier, fitter, stronger, sexier — and, oh yes, slimmer too, if that's what your body needs. Please understand that my philosophy isn't primarily about losing weight, but about being interested in eating good food and feeling really well. Just follow my plan and your body weight will regulate itself naturally. Believe me, I'm speaking from experience here. Now for those guides ...

GUIDE NUMBER ONE:
EAT AS MUCH FOOD AS YOU WANT UNTIL YOU ARE SATISFIED, AS LONG AS YOU EAT THE RIGHT FOODS PREPARED IN THE RIGHT WAY

The right foods are the simplest foods that grow from the earth in their most unadulterated, organic form — fresh vegetables, seasonal fruits, sprouted seeds, raw nuts and seeds, grains, beans, legumes, pulses — and certain vegetable proteins such as tofu together with some fish or organic turkey or chicken. It's what I call the "Diet of Abundance" — you'll find there are dozens of perfect foods you can eat all day long and feel great!

The recipes in this book will give you all the information you need on preparing these foods in the best way for optimum nutrition.

GUIDE NUMBER TWO:
NEVER GET FIXATED ON WEIGHT

If there's one thing I can teach you, it's that what you resist will persist. So if you become fixated on your weight, then you'll only make it a bigger issue for yourself. Ditch the weight issue. Forget it. It simply does not work. We've got more important things to do. Once you finally let the weight issue go, and adopt a new lifestyle plan, your body weight will regulate itself. Believe me, this is true.

In all my years in practice, I have never had to weigh a single client. Imagine that — a nutritionist consulting overweight clients who has no scales and doesn't ever weigh anyone. So don't forget: *you will get amazing results if you stop focusing on your weight and start focusing on eating the right foods.* Which brings me to ...

GUIDE NUMBER THREE:
DON'T DO FAD DIETS—THEY DON'T WORK IN THE LONG TERM

I've never seen a fad diet that really works in the long term. Some may work in the short term but all too often, once the dieter goes off their diet, they put the weight back on to an even greater extent than before. There's no end to the number and variations of these fad diets, and the problem I have with most of them is that they restrict too many different foods and food groups, leaving you nutritionally starved. Apart from anything else, some of them can cause a loss of essential fatty acids (EFAs)— which are actually needed for weight loss or weight management—mineral imbalances, vitamin deficiencies, gastric disturbances, and hormonal problems. My recipes, on the other hand, will help you get stronger and better nourished because I won't be cutting out what your body needs. And, as you now know, when you care about good health first, the weight issue will fall into place.

GUIDE NUMBER FOUR:
THIS IS A PLAN FOR LIFE

This simple philosophy needs to become second nature. To start with, you might want to carry this book into the supermarket or health food store to make the right purchasing choices; use this book in the kitchen at home for recipes; take it to work for referring to quick snacks; take it to restaurants for meal ideas. The *You Are What You Eat* concepts integrate and interconnect into every realm of your life. This is your route to wellness, happiness, and a great body.

GUIDE NUMBER FIVE:
IT'S GOT TO BE MY WAY OR THE HIGHWAY

Human health doesn't respond fully enough to half measures, so I want you to really go for it. It's not that I am some kind of perfectionist gone awry; I just want to make sure you have the best shot at feeling great. I know what shoddy health and excess weight feels like. I've been there. We've all been there. I know we can do far better together if you do what I tell you.

I remember a woman who came into my office for the first time. She was recovering from a very serious illness and wanted help with her nutrition.

I wanted so much for her to get well and felt that I could help her, but knew she would have to want it as much as me. As she walked in I greeted her with a warm smile. So far so good. Then she landed a large bottle of vodka on my desk with the immortal words, "I'll do your diet, darling, but I'm not giving up my vodka."

There was a deafening silence, then I walked to the door and opened it, saying, "You can leave now!"

She sat there, looking stunned, then blurted out, "Do you know who I am? My husband is world famous. We are very wealthy people."

So I gave her what-for: "Go back to your husband with your bottle of poison and drain him, but you're not going to drain me. I don't care who you are, who your husband is, what you do, or how much money you all have. It makes no difference to me. When it comes to health, we are one and the same. You are to leave now!"

I'd touched a nerve. She broke down into uncontrollable tears, sobbing bitterly, "I am desperate. Please help me. I'll do anything you say."

"Right," I said. "Take that bottle of alcohol and pour it down my office sink drain right now, and then we can get started."

And she did. And we got started. And she never looked back. She consulted with me for years. She became a new woman with a new body and with new heights of energy, hopes, and dreams.

For the next three months, I want you to eat according to my plan and recipes. After this first three-month period, you are welcome to introduce an 80:20 approach: do what I tell you 80 percent of the time and you can be naughty 20 percent of the time. So you see, things aren't so bad after all. But when you adopt my new ways, you may find that you enjoy the delicious taste of these healthy foods so much, and savor the feeling of wellness you have that you may not want to look back.

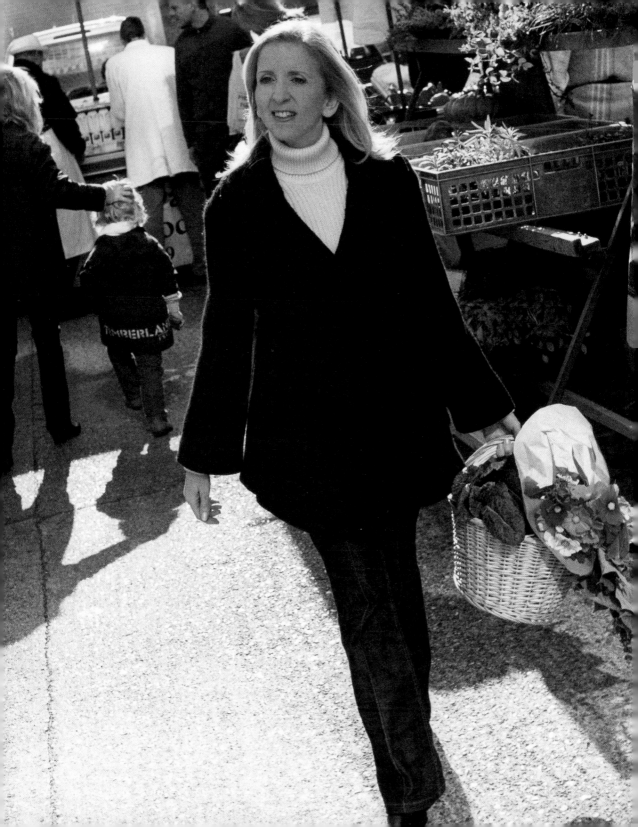

GUIDE NUMBER SIX:
BE CREATIVE AND PASSIONATE IN YOUR COOKING

What I want is to empower you to help yourself make the changes you need. This book will provide you with lots of ideas which I hope will not only keep you on the path to good health but also inspire you to create your own recipes.

Here's how it works. If you can make Hearty Lentil Stew (page 167), then you can make any stew. For example, you can change the lentils to kidney beans and the meal becomes a kidney bean stew. Change the kidney beans to chickpeas and it becomes a chickpea stew. Change the veggies, the herbs, and seasonings that go with the beans and voilà—you have a whole new set of food creations that you have developed yourself. This is empowerment.

GUIDE NUMBER SEVEN:
EMBRACE CHANGE

We can often be our own worst enemies when it comes to change: "I can't do this, I can't do that." We too often give ourselves continuous negative messages with constant restrictive limits. Here are just some of the things my TV participants have thrown at me:
"I don't like beans." (Before ever tasting them.)
"I hate the smell of brown rice."
"Millet looks gross."

The things we say to ourselves are listened to by our body at large. To involve yourself in my program, you will need to be open to new ideas, new foods, new ways. So don't get stuck in the mud. This is where you take responsibility for yourself. Get unstuck and get moving and you will be truly free to pursue your dreams, hopes, and goals for a deep, fulfilling life.

Ask yourself: What do I feel like eating today? Which bean, which herb, which veggies, which seasonings?

GUIDE NUMBER EIGHT:
BE IN TOUCH WITH YOUR EMOTIONS

After many years of working in the field of nutritional health, juggling work, family life, and everything else in between, I know from experience that it can be easy to lose yourself. I once had a client who was in her late forties and grossly overweight. She showed me photographs of herself taken nearly 25 years earlier, in which she looked wonderful: not only slim but sparkly-eyed and literally lit up with energy. I asked her what had happened and she explained that for over 20 years she had been eating junk food for comfort. Tears welled up in her eyes and, after gentle prompting, she slowly began to tell me how she had lost her baby daughter at just 22 days old. This woman had never been given counseling and had simply been using bad food to bury her pain for all that time. And it was only by opening up about her relationship with food that she had reached her most inner emotions, and realized how interconnected they had become.

I believe that our body, our emotions, and what we eat are all intricately linked. Each affects the other. This woman's experience may be rather more pronounced than the norm, but there is a general lesson for everyone here. In order to become a balanced, harmonious, and contented individual, and for your body to get the very best out of healthy food, you need to be in touch with yourself. Accept who you are. This is an important step toward being and staying healthy.

FOOD COMBINING MADE SIMPLE

The majority of the recipes in this book follow simple food combining rules. If you follow these guidelines, you may lose weight if you need to, and will do it simply and healthily. Plus you'll say good-bye to gas, bloating, and most digestive problems—and feel a million times better. However, once you have your weight and other diet-related issues resolved then you won't need to be quite so strict. It's still best to follow my guidelines as much as you can, though, as it's a sure path to feeling fantastic.

A more detailed explanation of food combining is in my previous book *You Are What You Eat*, but in very simple terms this is what you need to know:

GROUP 1: PROTEINS
- Cheese
- Eggs
- Fish
- Game/rabbit
- Meat
- Milk
- Nuts
- Poultry
- Shellfish
- Soybeans, tofu, and soy products
- Yogurt

GROUP 2: CARBOHYDRATES
- Grains: including oats, pasta, rice, rye, corn, millet
- Grain products: including cookies, bread, cakes, crackers, pastries
- Honey
- Maple syrup
- Starchy vegetables: including potatoes, yams, and corn
- Sugar and sweets

GROUP 3: NON-STARCHY VEGETABLES AND FATS
- Butter, cream
- Herbs, spices, seasonings
- Olive and other oils
- Salads and leafy greens
- Seeds

GROUP 4: FRUIT
- All varieties

FOOD COMBINING CHART

YES

- ▻ Groups 1 and 3
- ▻ Groups 2 and 3
- ▻ Group 4 alone

NO

- ▻ Groups 1 and 2
- ▻ Groups 1 and 4
- ▻ Groups 2 and 4
- ▻ Groups 3 and 4

TIPS ON FOOD COMBINING

- ▻ Always eat fruit by itself, 30 minutes before other food groups and, ideally, first thing in the morning on an empty stomach.
- ▻ Leave two hours after a carbohydrate meal before eating a dense protein meal.
- ▻ Leave three hours after a protein meal before eating carbohydrates.
- ▻ Beans and pulses have a mixture of starch and protein, predominantly starch. You can combine most pulses and beans with grains as well as salads and vegetables.

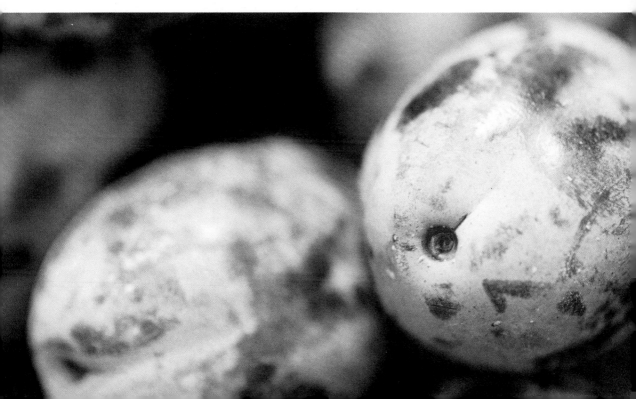

BODY CHECK

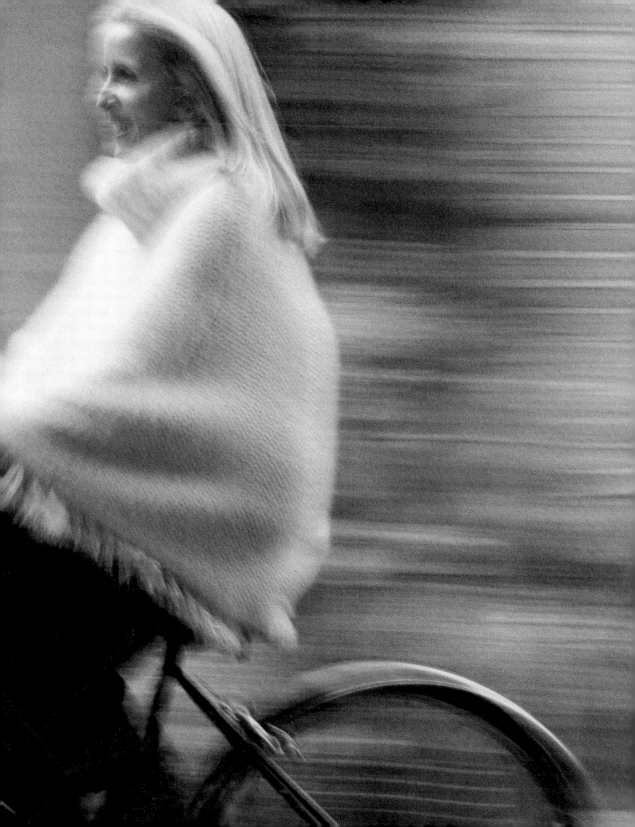

ALL THE RECIPES IN THIS BOOK ARE SIMPLY VERY GOOD FOR YOU. HOWEVER, IT'S ALSO GREAT TO HAVE A SENSE OF JUST HOW HEALTHY, OR PERHAPS I SHOULD SAY UNHEALTHY, YOU ARE. IN THE ORIGINAL BOOK *YOU ARE WHAT YOU EAT* I INCLUDED A BIG CHAPTER ON GETTING TO KNOW YOUR BODY. HERE I'VE INCLUDED A QUICK QUESTIONNAIRE THAT WILL GIVE YOU A GOOD IDEA OF HOW YOU'RE DOING ON THE McKEITH SCALE OF HEALTHY LIVING. SOME OF MY QUESTIONS ARE QUITE SPECIFIC TO HELP YOU WITH YOUR BODY CHECK; PERHAPS YOU'RE MEGA STRESSED, OR YOU NEED TO DETOX. IF THAT'S THE CASE I'LL POINT YOU IN THE DIRECTION OF SOME GREAT RECIPES WHICH ARE PERFECT FOR YOU. AS ALWAYS, I ADVISE THAT IF YOU ARE CONSIDERING A RADICAL CHANGE OF DIET, YOU SHOULD CONSULT YOUR GP FIRST—ESPECIALLY IF YOU ARE PREGNANT, ELDERLY, OR UNDER 16.

GETTING TO GRIPS WITH YOU: McKEITH DIET CHECK

All of my clients are required to keep a record of everything that they eat and drink for a week. I recommend that you do the same. You may surprise yourself and learn a lot about your habits. You just might see that you are not eating as well as you had convinced yourself or that you may be eating the same things every day. Alternatively, you may find out that things are actually looking good. Either way, you will be more aware of yourself and what you put into your body.

ANSWER THE FOLLOWING QUESTIONS WITH A YES OR NO:

1. Do you drink a minimum of 2 quarts of still (mineral or filtered) water a day?
2. Do you eat fresh fruit and vegetables every day?
3. Do you eat essential fats in the form of fish, avocados, nuts, seeds, or cold-pressed oils on a regular basis every week?
4. Do you avoid foods containing preservatives, additives, sugar, and salt?
5. Do you cook from scratch rather than using cans and packets?
6. Do you eat a range of whole grains such as millet, oats, brown rice, rye, quinoa, and barley, rather than white, refined grains?
7. Do you eat a non-sugary breakfast every day?
8. Do you eat pulses, such as chickpeas, beans, and lentils at least 3 times a week or more?
9. Do you choose organically grown foods where possible?
10. Do you avoid fizzy drinks, caffeinated tea, coffee, and alcohol?
11. Do you eat a healthy lunch each day?
12. Do you eat a healthy dinner before 7:30 p.m. each day?

ADD UP YOUR YES ANSWERS. THIS IS YOUR SCORE.

▶ **10 or more**
YOU ARE LIKE A DR. GILLIAN GROUPIE!
You are definitely in my "good books." I am proud of you, so well done! It looks like you are really making an effort. You and your body will benefit now and in the future so please keep it up. You're going to get a real buzz from my Veggie Vitality Juice (page 53) and I hope you discover lots of new recipes in this book which you might not have tried before. The key for you is to keep your healthy food choices as varied as possible for ultimate nutrition.

▶ **Between 6 and 9**
COULD TRY HARDER
When it comes to your body and good health, you know that I believe half-measures to be unacceptable, and you should feel this too. The bottom line is that you probably don't feel 100 percent, so either do it right or not at all. Get on track now. You'll be happier, with a much healthier body and a far sexier one too. You'll thank me for it. I'm sure you're no stranger to lettuce, but perhaps you need some more exciting ideas—check out Crunchy Walnut Coleslaw (page 111), Tabbouleh (page 114), or even my Seaweed Salad (page 124). And if you need a bit of convincing that beans are far from boring, try the Adzuki Bean Stew (page 158) with Onion Gravy (page 229). Top it with my healthy Millet Mash (page 159).
Go for it.

ON A SLIPPERY SLOPE

I doubt you are even close to experiencing optimum health and vitality. I urge you to start out with the smoothies and take each day at a time. You will love my Mango Mania (page 61). Once you have tried that, you will be hooked. Also try the Quick Bites (pages 186–199), which don't take much time at all. Just think how different things could be if you allowed yourself to be McKeith'd. Read the Food Philosophy chapter, specifically the section

Embrace Change (page 14). As a special treat to get started, get a friend or a loved one to make one of my recipes for you. I have found that for people who are finding the transition from an unhealthy to healthy diet difficult my Chicken Burgers (page 136) with Raw Salsa (page 210) and a crunchy green salad of snowpeas, fennel, celery, carrots, and beets are perfect. Shepherdess Pie (page 141) is our family favorite. Some very easy changes will make a huge difference. So take that important first step.

IMMUNE SYSTEM CHECK

The foods you eat are like a tonic to the immune system. Certain foods can suppress immune function while the right foods may actually boost immune activity. For example, sprouted broccoli seeds have been shown to be one of the most powerful immune-boosting foods that we know of. Conversely, people who eat high quantities of foods with refined sugars often suffer from allergies, food intolerances, chemical sensitivities, hay fever, colds, flu, headaches, and other disorders, all of which are related to immune dysfunction. In our modern world, immune degradation is becoming a prevalent issue among the mass population at large.

ANSWER YES OR NO:

1. Do you have bad breath?
2. Do you suffer from congestion or a runny nose?
3. Does your tongue have a thick white or yellow coating or teeth marks around the side?
4. Do you have dark circles under your eyes?
5. Do you have white spots on your nails?
6. Do you have pain or sensitivity under the right rib area?
7. Do you have thrush or yeast problems?
8. Are you tired all the time?
9. Do you catch colds or the flu frequently?
10. Do you suffer from hayfever, allergies, or food sensitivities?

ADD UP YOUR YES ANSWERS TO FIND OUT YOUR SCORE.

▶ **Between 7 and 10**
IMMUNE BASKETCASE

You urgently need to comply with everything that I tell you. Do not miss my Carrot and Almond Soup (page 83), which is a really easy place to start. Carrots are high in the antioxidant beta-carotene and vitamins A and D. Eat sprouted seeds (page 35) and get into fruit because of the high vitamin content. Pineapple is a great source of vitamin C, for example. Grilled Banana with Citrus Spice (page 221) is a delicious fruit treat and for breakfast, road test my fruit salads (page 71). If you feel the onset of a cold or the flu, try using cinnamon in your juices and smoothies (pages 50–66), or in herbal teas (pages 40–41). Cinnamon has a historical use of providing relief when faced with these symptoms, especially when mixed in a tea with some fresh ginger.

▶ **Between 4 and 6**
MESS WAITING TO HAPPEN

Act before it's too late. Whenever you feel under par, make a Sprout Surprise Juice (page 54). You will love my immune boosting Baked Salmon with Spinach and Leeks (page 146). There's lots of fresh ginger in this dish, which is beneficial for the immune system, and spinach, which is a good source of another immune booster, CoQ10. This recipe also has lots of onions—it's important to eat lots of onions (and garlic). I once had a friend who worked in an onion and garlic factory. He said that in the entire time he worked in the onion job, he never once had a cold! Several anti-inflammatory agents in onions render them helpful with the respiratory congestion associated with the common cold. Both onions and garlic also contain compounds that may help reduce inflammation. In addition, the quercitin and other flavonoids found in onions work with vitamin C to help kill harmful bacteria, making onions an especially good addition to soups and stews during cold and flu season.

▶ **Between 1 and 3**
HOPEFUL

There's still a little work to be done, but you could lift yourself up fairly quickly. You too should eat lots of powerful sprouted broccoli seeds whenever you get the chance. And start growing your own sprouted seeds too. Commit to making 2–3 vegetable juices (pages 52–57) every week, thus delivering lots of nutrients to your immune system. I have a client who used to live on chips and burgers and now her favorite recipe is the Fennel Fun Juice (page 57). Also, try my Sea Vegetable and Sprout Salad (page 116) and don't miss out on the immune boosting Raw Avocado and Cucumber Soup (page 96).

TOXIN CHECK

Some people treat themselves like a toxic waste dump, loading themselves with unhealthy food choices that are difficult to digest. This creates toxins. Such toxins may strip the body of much needed nutrients. You end up feeling like a dishrag.

ARE YOU A TOXIC LOADER?

1. Do you add table salt to your cooking and/or to food before you have even tasted it?
2. Do you add sugar to your tea or coffee?
3. Do you drink caffeinated tea, coffee, tap water, diet drinks, or fizzy drinks regularly?
4. Do you eat packaged foods laden with preservatives or chemicals that you cannot pronounce?
5. Do you eat such processed, packaged, or microwaveable meals more than 3 times weekly?
6. Do you drink more than the recommended amount of alcohol every week or binge drink on weekends?
7. Are you a takeout junkie?
8. Do you suffer from constant headaches?
9. Do you have spots or acne anywhere on your skin or do you suffer from hives or have hemorrhoids?
10. Do you smoke cigarettes or use recreational drugs?

HOW MUCH ALCOHOL IS TOO MUCH?

The medically recommended units of alcohol per week is 14 for women and 21 for men. One unit of alcohol is 10 ml (about 1/3 ounce) by volume, or 8 g (.3 ounce) by weight, of pure alcohol. For example: A half-pint of average strength beer, cider, or lager (4–5% alcohol by volume) contains 1 unit. A small pub measure (25 ml or about 1 ounce) of spirits (40% alcohol by volume) contains 1 unit. A standard pub measure (35 ml or about 1 1/4 ounces) of spirits contains 1 1/2 units. A small glass (125ml or about 1/2 cup) of average strength wine (12% alcohol by volume) contains 1 1/2 units.

ADD UP YOUR YES ANSWERS TO FIND OUT YOUR SCORE.

▶ **Between 8 and 10**
EXIT 13 TOXIC WASTE DUMP*
If you continue down this route, you might as well take the exit right now because I can't help you. You had better either do it my way or it's the highway for you. The first thing you must do is make my simple and detoxifying Veggie Virgin Juice (page 52). It tastes delicious, absolutely scrumptious. But to truly get on the detox drive, you cannot miss the Mung Bean Casserole (page 183) with Gourmet Brown Rice (page 195) and a crunchy salad. It's the best dish ever for ridding the body of nasty toxins and bacteria. So many of the TV participants have told me how this recipe has put them on the road to healthy eating. If they can do it, you can too.

▶ **Between 5 and 7**
PRETTY PUTRID
Start juicing my vegetable concoctions right away, especially Fennel Fun (page 57) and Total Cleanser (page 51) to give you a cleanout. This is the most incredible detoxification tonic.

▶ **Between 2 and 4**
TOXIC TEASER
You are teetering in either direction. Instead of going downhill, keep going in my direction. Turn on to crunchy salads (pages 109–126), as you need lots of food enzymes. Toxic types are often deficient in good, healthy essential fats and minerals. Redress the balance with a big Green Salad (page 124) and also try the Spring Salad (page 113), a fantastic source of essential fats.

(*Exit 13 on the New Jersey Turnpike is the most toxic place on earth as far as I'm concerned!)

THE TONGUE CHECK

Your tongue is a very telling indicator of how healthy your diet is.

1. Does your tongue have a line down the middle?
2. Does you tongue have teeth marks round the side?
3. Does you tongue have a bright red tip?
4. Is your tongue sore?
5. Does you tongue appear dotted all over?

IF YOU ANSWER YES TO A PARTICULAR QUESTION, IT COULD MEAN:

1. Weak digestion. You may feel bloated and suffer from gas or indigestion. A strong digestive system is important for nutrient absorption. I would suggest food combining for a period of eight weeks (see pages 16–17). Keep meals simple, and ingredients that are particularly good for you include brown rice, avocado, and tofu. Try the Avocado and Barley Salad (page 109), Smoked Tofu and Bean Burgers (page 155), Tofu with Steamed Vegetables (page 177), and Gourmet Brown Rice (page 195).

2. Spleen weakness and nutrient deficiencies. Your spleen is your energy battery and may not be taking up nutrients as effectively as it should. Symptoms can include feeling tired all the time, gassy, and bloated. Adzuki Bean Stew (page 158) is a good digestion strengthener, so don't miss out on this. And look for recipes that contain beets (page 86), celery, fennel (page 57), dill (page 167), chicken (page 139), garlic, kidney beans (page 180), parsley (page 114), pumpkins (page 88), and turnips (page 85).

3. A red tip may indicate either emotional upset or that your body is stressed. Either way, you will need B vitamins to calm it all down. Foods rich in B vitamins include brown rice and other whole grains, root vegetables, and beans. Go for my Navy Bean Loaf (page 144), Mediterranean Black-Eyed Pea Casserole (page 145), Chickpea Burgers (page 135), and Gourmet Brown Rice (page 195).

4. A sore tongue may indicate a vitamin B_6 deficiency, and could also indicate that niacin and/or iron levels are low. Drink nettle or dandelion teas (pages 40–41) and eat foods rich in vitamin B_6, including sunflower seeds, brown rice, buckwheat, and avocados. Try my Juicy Smoothie (page 66), Tabbouleh (page 114), and breakfast porridges (pages 75–76). Best-Ever Beet Soup (page 86) should regularly be on the menu in your house too.

5. This can be a sign of what I call liver stagnation. In Western holistic medicine, we think of the liver as the organ of detoxification. The liver tries to keep toxins out of your bloodstream, particularly those come into your body via your diet. When your liver is overworked, it may perform sluggishly. In the West this is often called a congested liver. Foods that support the liver are good for everyone, and include cruciferous veggies such as kohlrabi (page 111), broccoli (page 125), cauliflower (page 104), flax seeds (page 75), hemp seeds (page 88), and sunflower seeds. Nettle and dandelion teas help too (page 40). White Bean and Cabbage Soup is a must (page 90).

GETTING ORGANIZED

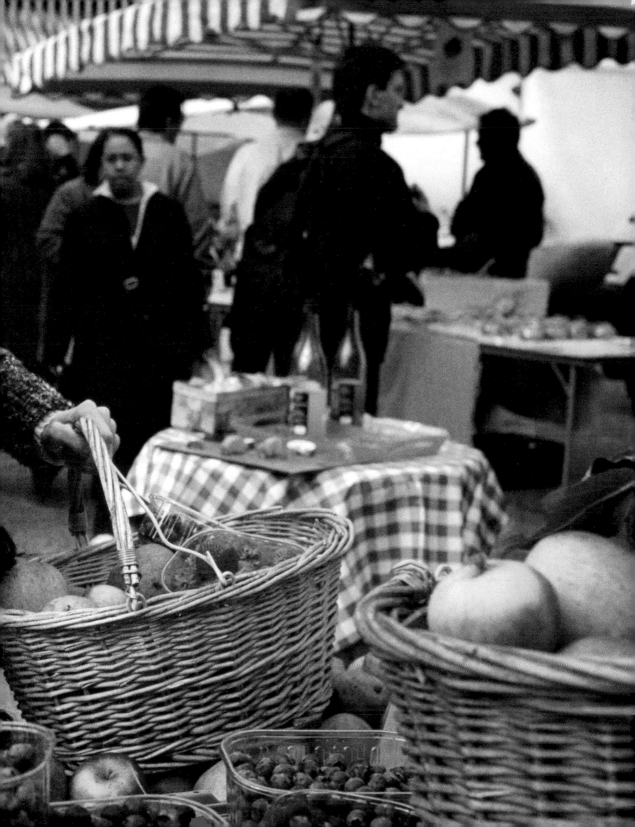

10 STEPS TO GET IT TOGETHER

When you're struggling to cope with a hectic job, a home, and a family, organization is the key. I once learned a hard lesson about being organized. Here's how it goes . . .

Years ago, when I was a student, my friend and I left the house one afternoon, and returned to find the front door ajar. Afraid we'd been burgled—and terrified that the burglar was still in the house—we called the police, who came to our rescue. One of the constables ran into the house and came out moments later with the words, "Miss, the good news is that there's no one in your house right now. But the bad news, I'm sorry to say, is that the house has been ransacked. It's totally vandalized—the burglars have done a real number on it." Another officer asked if I had any enemies—someone who wanted to hurt me (an old boyfriend, perhaps?), but I couldn't think of anyone.

I felt invaded, violated, and angry. There's nothing worse than the feeling of your own home being burgled and destroyed. The police suggested that they walk me through the premises to identify the damages and stolen goods. We started with the kitchen, which they said had been the worst hit. I walked into the room with them, and slowly took in the situation. "Oh dear," I said. "Everything seems to still be here."

It was so embarrassing. Nothing had been stolen. Absolutely nothing. The mess that surrounded me had nothing to do with burglars; this was just the way I kept my kitchen back then. A bloody mess!

From that moment on, I vowed to get my life in order, and I started with the kitchen. Here are my 10 steps to get it together:

1. KEEP A TIDY KITCHEN

The kitchen represents the focal point of the home and the center of our lives—after all, it's here that we feed our bodies with fuel to thrive. And since food is a major component of life, the kitchen is a critical space in the house, or at least it should be. A tidy kitchen means a tidy mind, a tidy body, and a tidy you. Get your kitchen in order and you will soon find your whole life follows suit. OK, so maybe you think I am overstating this. But I want you to go and get your kitchen in order. Today! Get rid of all that rubbish, including those useless papers, tape dispensers, paper clips, old birthday cards, and more that you've been hoarding in that drawer. Just do it, and see the difference in your home, your mind, and your life. It's a great start to everything we need to do together here.

2. GET RID OF JUNK FOODS

The first step toward healthy eating is choosing healthy ingredients. Start by throwing out salty convenience foods, fatty foods, sugary drinks, chemical snacks, foods with unpronounceable ingredients you can't decipher, hydrogenated oils, and processed junk food from your fridge and cabinets.

3. SHOP IN THE RIGHT FRAME OF MIND

Never shop when you're hungry—you'll end up loading your cart with sugar-rich but nutrient-poor convenience foods such as pies, chips, candy, cakes, and cookies, all of which should be limited on a healthy eating plan. Have a clear idea of what you are going to eat and the ingredients you need—you'll be less likely to make unhealthy choices. Take this book with you if it helps—that way you'll have quick and easy access to my recipes and their ingredients. It'll be as if I'm with you, helping you out!

4. CHANGE YOUR SNACK MIND-SET

Stop thinking of quick snacks as sugary granola bars, cookies, chocolates, chips and other nasties. Start associating fast, on-the-run snacks with easy, healthy alternatives. In the morning, for example, grab a couple of whole peppers, a whole cucumber, and a celery stick. Wash them, throw them in a bag, and voilà, you have your morning and afternoon snacks for the day. Eat the pepper whole, in the same way as you would an apple. Just hold it in your hand and bite into it. This is the new way of snacking with whole vegetables—you don't have to spend all that time and energy slicing them. It's faster, easier, and healthier. See chapter 10 for lots of easy snack recipes and ideas (pages 200–213).

5. MAKE GOOD USE OF YOUR FRIDGE/FREEZER

Make sure you know how to make the most of your freezer. Did you, for example, know that you can freeze fresh herbs? Or that freezing grains will prevent mold and critters from taking over them? Think of your freezer as a form of natural preservative. Keep your perishables in there and bring them out to the larder or fridge on the week you want to use them.

Most fridge-freezers are the size of postage stamps and are usually at feet level. Half the time you can't get down there to see what's in them unless you have a good back, strong knees, and exceptional eyesight. So, if you ever have any spare cash, go out and buy the biggest fridge-freezer you can find.

6. STOCK UP ON KITCHEN EQUIPMENT

While traveling the country with the TV series *You Are What You Eat*, I've noticed that most people don't have enough basic items of kitchen equipment, such as sharp knives, or a good range of pots, plates, and mixing bowls.

HERE'S MY LIST OF KITCHEN EQUIPMENT ESSENTIALS:

- ► baking sheets
- ► large casserole dish
- ► measuring cup
- ► metal grater
- ► peeler
- ► plastic cutting board for fish
- ► scale
- ► set of saucepans
- ► set of sharp knives
- ► thick wooden cutting board
- ► wok
- ► wooden spoons

SOME EXTRA MUST-HAVES

When you have these items, the sky's the limit with how creative you can be:

- ► food processor (apart from everything else, it will blend, whisk, and turn nuts into a fluffy whipped cream)
- ► blender (for your morning fruit smoothies and blended smooth soups)
- ► juicer (for your fruit or vegetable juices)
- ► And if you really want to treat yourself, buy a spiralizer. This is my most recent kitchen discovery and I love it. It's an amazing gadget that can make delicious raw spaghetti from any root vegetable. Sounds crazy, but when you apply it to butternut squash, beets, or sweet potatoes, you end up with a food that tastes like spaghetti, looks like spaghetti, and has a similar consistency and texture to spaghetti. It's almost hard to believe that you are not eating pasta but in fact raw root vegetables full of food enzymes. Your kids will just gobble up this new form of uncooked pasta without the refined flour of regular white pasta.

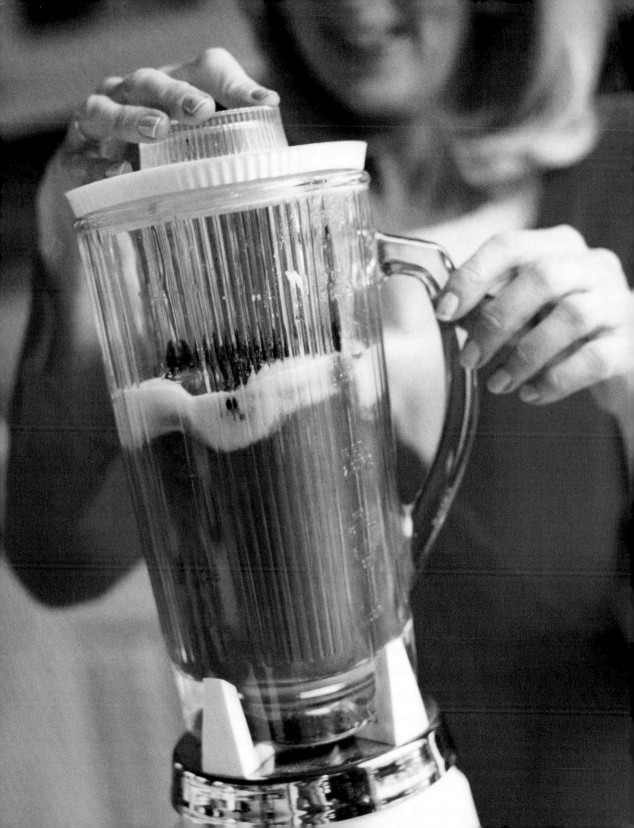

7. DON'T BE AFRAID OF HEALTH FOOD STORES

Years ago, when I was a student at Edinburgh University, I had a boyfriend who was a health food junkie. I thought he was a bit strange in those days eating tofu (instead of meat), bean chips (instead of potato chips), and blackstrap molasses (instead of sugar). But it must have been working in his favor: his body was in impeccable condition. He's the one who first introduced me to the world of health food stores and got me hooked.

Health food stores generally tend to be the pioneers for many products that eventually make their way onto supermarket shelves. This was exactly what happened with yogurt, for example. When it first came onto the market years ago, it was only available in health food stores, but over time it proved to be a big seller, and began to be stocked by supermarkets. It was exactly the same with brown rice, tofu, rice milk, and even soy sauce.

My point here is that you need not fear health food stores. It's true, when you first go into one many of the foods may seem strange and unusual. But, remember, many of those weird-sounding foods could soon become the regular foods that we all buy from the supermarket.

Health food stores often stock healthy alternatives to conventional products; for example, cookies with no added sugar, or healthy alternatives to meat and animal proteins, such as tofu and tempeh. I've even found alternative juice drinks sweetened with apple juice instead of sugar; sugar-free corn flakes; salt-free vegetable bouillon powders for making soups; bouquets of dried powdered herb seasonings as salt alternatives, and so on.

Health food stores pride themselves on carrying products that are healthy, organic, and contain no chemicals, no preservatives, and no artificial ingredients. They carry many products with particular health benefits such as sea vegetables or seaweeds, beans, grains, pulses, seeds and nuts, vitamin, mineral, and superfood supplements, and herb teas. So have no fear, health foods are here!

8. FOLLOW THESE HEALTHY SHOPPING GUIDELINES

The major supermarkets should have at least 90 percent or more of the foods mentioned here. You can also fill in at farmers' markets and health food stores or websites (www.gillianmckeith.com).

▶ Load up on fresh fruits, vegetables, and sprouted seeds.

▶ Buy fresh fish—preferably white or oily. If you must eat red meat, buy fresh, organic lean meat, which is much more nutritious than sausages and processed meats.

▶ Avoid fruit juices made with sugar and preservatives and go for fresh, unsweetened juices instead.

▶ When buying dairy products, go for natural yogurt and even try grain milks such as spelt milk, almond milk, amaranth milk, oat milk or rice milk, for a change.

▶ Choose softer cheeses such as goat cheese, cottage cheese, and ricotta instead of hard cheeses.

▶ Avoid packaged meals, convenience foods, and canned foods containing salt, sugar, and preservatives. They are likely to be low in nutrients and high in calories, additives, and chemicals. Read the labels first.

Oily fish are rich in omega-3 fats,
the "good" fats.

9. STOCK UP ON STAPLES

The following items are pantry essentials and staples for your kitchen. Most of them are available in supermarkets or health food stores.

▶ DRIED HERBS

I love fresh herbs most of all and use them liberally in my cooking and salads (see page 38). But dried herbs can come in handy for seasoning too. Buy the following organic dried herbs:

- ▶ Basil
- ▶ Bay leaves
- ▶ Dill
- ▶ Fennel
- ▶ Fenugreek
- ▶ Garlic
- ▶ Mint
- ▶ Oregano
- ▶ Rosemary
- ▶ Tarragon
- ▶ Thyme

▶ SPICES

- ▶ Cinnamon (ground)
- ▶ Cloves
- ▶ Coriander seeds
- ▶ Cumin (ground)
- ▶ Ginger
- ▶ Mustard seeds
- ▶ Nutmeg
- ▶ Saffron
- ▶ Turmeric

▶ FLAVORINGS (SAVORY)

- ▶ Agar-agar flakes (neutral-tasting seaweed which provides jelly-like consistency— perfect for healthy desserts)
- ▶ Almond powder
- ▶ Bouillon powder or vegetable stock cubes
- ▶ Brown rice vinegar
- ▶ Capers
- ▶ Cider vinegar
- ▶ Mirin
- ▶ Miso paste (a fantastic way to flavor foods— try all the different types, from the meaty hatcho miso to the lighter white misos)
- ▶ Nori flakes
- ▶ Seaweed flake seasonings
- ▶ Seaweeds
- ▶ Sesame sauce
- ▶ Shoyu soy sauce
- ▶ Tahini
- ▶ Tamari (wheat-free soy) sauce
- ▶ Umeboshi paste
- ▶ Umeboshi plum seasoning

▶ FLAVORINGS (SWEET)

- ▶ Apple juice
- ▶ Barley malt syrup
- ▶ Brown rice syrup
- ▶ Carob powder
- ▶ Date syrup or date paste (you can make your own date paste by blending fresh dates and water together in the blender)
- ▶ Grain milks (rice, soy, oat, spelt, amaranth, millet, and almond)
- ▶ Maple syrup
- ▶ Vanilla bean
- ▶ Vanilla extract

NUTS AND SEEDS

Nuts and seeds are power-packed with nutrients and healthy, good fats. They are best eaten in moderation, but I thoroughly recommend a small handful as a snack. Alternatively, sprinkle them whole on cereals or chopped on salads and soups. Because of their high fat content, nuts and seeds keep at room temperature for only about a month (in an airtight container in dark, cool cupboard), but will keep for four months in the fridge and eight months in the freezer. If you find nuts hard to digest, try soaking them in water overnight.

- Almonds
- Brazil nuts
- Cashews
- Chestnuts
- Hazelnuts
- Pecans
- Pine nuts
- Pistachios
- Walnuts
- Flax seeds
- Hemp seeds
- Pumpkin seeds
- Sesame seeds
- Sunflower seeds

SPROUTED SEEDS

Sprouts are nutritional stars. They are fantastic immunity boosters, being high in antioxidants, vitamins, minerals, protein, enzymes and fiber. You can buy them in health food stores or even try sprouting your own (see my previous book, *You Are What You Eat*). Always eat these sprouts raw, whether in salads or added to hot savory dishes just before serving.

- Alfalfa sprouts
- Broccoli seed sprouts
- Clover seed sprouts
- Lentil sprouts
- Mung bean sprouts

OILS

Always get cold-pressed nut and seed oils.

- Avocado
- Hemp
- Olive
- Pumpkin seed
- Sesame
- Sunflower
- Walnut

BEANS AND PULSES

Beans are rich in essential nutrients, high in fiber, and are a source of good, healthy fats. Research has shown that a regular intake of beans can help lower cholesterol levels and the risks of heart attack, and may help inhibit the growth of cancer cells. Beans are a very good source of protein, but with the exception of soybeans (which are a complete protein), they need to be eaten with grains to form a complete protein that the body can readily absorb. Beans are incredibly versatile when it comes to creating recipes, and I am a huge fan. Store dried beans in an airtight container at room temperature and they will keep almost indefinitely. Keep fresh beans in perforated plastic bags in the fridge crisper section; edible pod beans will keep for three to five days, shell beans for two to three days.

- Adzukis
- Black beans
- Black-eyed peas
- Fava beans
- Cannellini beans
- Chickpeas
- Flageolets
- Navy beans
- Kidney beans
- Lentils
- Lima beans
- Mung beans
- Soybeans
- Split peas

▶ TEMPEH

You'll find tempeh in health food stores in the fridge section. Made from soybeans, tempeh provides a good supply of B vitamins. It's a very nutritious substitute for meat.

▶ TOFU

Try the different types. The silky soft one is great for sauces; the firmer ones are best for snacks or stews.

▶ MISO

Miso is a fermented soybean paste and is packed with immune-supporting minerals and energy-boosting B vitamins. You can find it in paste or powder form in health food stores and it's a valuable addition to your kitchen cupboard. There are many varieties, ranging from light to dark, a taste for every palate. Try my Ten-Minute Miso Fish Soup (page 93) for an instant pick-me-up.

▶ FLOURS

You won't need all these flours but it's good to know what's out there. Just pick one or two.

- ▶ Hemp
- ▶ Millet
- ▶ Oat
- ▶ Potato
- ▶ Quinoa
- ▶ Rice
- ▶ Soy
- ▶ Sunflower seed
- ▶ Whole-wheat

▶ GRAINS

Grains are your basic energy food. I always recommend unrefined grains, which are not only a good source of complex carbohydrates, but also fiber, B vitamins, vitamin E, calcium, magnesium, potassium, iron, zinc, copper, and selenium. Research shows that a diet rich in unrefined grains can help lower cholesterol and regulate blood sugar levels. Grains provide the perfect accompaniment to all my bean dishes, and they make delicious and fulfilling meals out of salads. Store whole grains in airtight containers away from heat, light, and moisture. Different grains have different storage times, so be sure to check. You can store grains for longer in the fridge or freezer.

- ▶ Amaranth
- ▶ Barley
- ▶ Brown Basmati rice
- ▶ Brown rice
- ▶ Buckwheat
- ▶ Bulgar
- ▶ Couscous
- ▶ Millet
- ▶ Oats
- ▶ Spelt
- ▶ Quinoa

▶ FRUIT

Fruits are packed with nutrients. Eat a wide variety of fruits to ensure a variety of goodness, from the B vitamins, folate, and potassium in bananas (a nutritious energy boost alternative to sweets) to the high levels of vitamin C in citrus fruits such as lemons and limes. Dried fruits like dates and figs are a good source of fiber (and a yummy snack), while dark orange fruits (apricots, peaches, and mangoes) are rich in antioxidants. Far and away the nutrient winners are the berry fruits, including strawberries, raspberries, blackberries, blueberries, cherries, and cranberries. Berries are rich in bioflavonoids, which have powerful antioxidant, anti-infective, and anti-inflammatory properties. They literally help the body to resist illness. Remember that it's not a good idea to combine fruit with other food groups (see page 17). It's an excellent idea to eat just one type of fruit, for example a bowl of blueberries or raspberries. But also try out my fab fruit salads (page 71).

VEGETABLES

Eat lots of dark green leafy vegetables, such as kale, cabbage, or broccoli, and alliums, such as garlic, onions, or leeks, at least once a day. Fresh, raw vegetables are rich in phytochemicals, which can be beneficial to your heart, skin, hair, mental, reproductive, and overall health. Eat lots of the following vegetables.

- Arugula
- Asparagus
- Broccoli
- Cabbage
- Carrots
- Cauliflower
- Celery
- Garlic
- Kale
- Leeks
- Mustard greens
- Onions
- Parsley
- Peas (green)
- Peppers
- Romaine lettuce
- Spinach
- Sweet potatoes
- Tomatoes
- Turnip greens
- Turnips
- Watercress
- Yams

SUPERFOOD SUPPLEMENTS

It might be a good idea to add a multi-vitamin and mineral supplement to your shopping basket to help correct nutritional deficiencies and protect against the nutrient-depleting effects of stress, poor diet, and environmental toxins. Following are the key supplements I would recommend that you take every day for constitutional support.

SUPPLEMENT BASKET

My supplement basket often consists of green superfoods as follows:

- Liquid algae (which I squirt into my mouth because it's like a nutrient shot of minerals)
- Spirulina tablets or powder for my smoothies
- Gillian McKeith's Organic Energy Powder formulation for a complete nutritional foundation (use in smoothies too)
- Aloe vera juice for healthy bowels and digestive tract (preferably non-bitter)

10. COOK IN THE RAW

I always advise my clients to include raw foods in the same meal when they prepare cooked foods. This is because raw foods contain food enzymes that are essential for optimum digestion and general well-being. Adding raw vegetables, raw seeds, or raw nuts is a great way of taking in food enzymes. Just think of them as "Digestive Dynamos."

HERBS

Herbs make truly fantastic natural flavorings—you won't miss salt if
you use them! Be passionate. Feel free to use generous proportions when
using them in cooking. Experiment to your heart's content and discover
your true favorites. Most herbs have healing properties, and these green
plants also contain an abundance of minerals, so you'll see lots used
in my recipes. Here are some of my favorite herbs:

BASIL

Basil has a cooling quality, which
means it can help to neutralize harmful
acids in the gut. This sweet-tasting herb
has been used for years as a calming
aid for indigestion. It tastes great
in salads. My favorite!

BAY

Bay leaves add great flavor to soups,
stews, sauces, and stock (but remember
not to actually eat them). They are
also thought to help with gas, headaches,
and indigestion.

CHERVIL

Chervil has a unique flavor that's a
little like parsley with a hint of aniseed.
It is thought to help stimulate and
ease digestion. It has such a wonderful
flavor that it can take a simple dish
and turn it into a gourmet delicacy.

CHIVES

Numerous studies have linked plants
like chives to helping lower and prevent
hypertension. Chives are also rich in
vitamin C and iron. Chives are the
perfect companion to cucumber
(see page 96 for my Avocado and
Cucumber Soup).

CILANTRO

In herbalism, cilantro is known
as an "alterative," which simply means
it can help purify the blood. Cilantro
also helps the body absorb nutrients
and remove waste matter. I often
add cilantro to recipes that include
beans because of its ability to
assist digestion.

DILL

Dill is a warming herb and a good
source of fiber, iron, magnesium, and
calcium. Another top choice for me.
It can be strengthening to the spleen,
liver, and stomach organs. I use dill
in salads, soups, casseroles, and even
in my Hearty Lentil Stew (see page 167).
It works like a charm.

LOVAGE

I love this herb. Its aromatic elements are similar to those in celery and it will add real zip to your dishes. It's also a diuretic and thus a good addition to any weight-loss program. Lovage is great simply thrown into any soup just before serving.

OREGANO

Oregano has an antioxidant punch (remember, antioxidants are powerful allies in helping to prevent cancer, heart disease, and stroke). Its antioxidant properties are partly due to the presence of rosmarinic acid, an antibacterial, antiviral, and antioxidant compound. Oregano goes wonderfully well with tomatoes so it's perfect for marinades, stews, and tomato sauces.

PARSLEY

Parsley is the culinary multivitamin, a nutrient powerhouse. It is a good source of beta-carotene, calcium, and more vitamin C than citrus fruits. This is one of the most important plants for providing vitamins to the body. It helps the body's defensive mechanisms and this may help keep negative bacteria at bay. If you warm parsley slightly, its flavor will soften and adapt nicely to whatever food you are preparing, so you can use this herb in just about any savory dish. It's very nourishing and restoring, and can help neutralize the intense flavor of garlic on the breath.

ROSEMARY

Rosemary contains properties that can help support the immune system. It's also thought to increase blood flow to the head and brain, increasing concentration and improving memory. I love to add a few sprigs while roasting vegetables, but remember not to eat the twigs.

TARRAGON

This strong aniseed-perfumed herb contains compounds that are believed to help lower blood pressure. When added to a dish it's best used in moderation because of the intense flavor, but it's delicious with chicken or fish, and in stews.

THYME

Thyme is considered a healing herb and is particularly good for chest and respiratory problems. It has antiseptic properties too. So adding fresh thyme to your salad dressing not only enhances flavor but also adds nutrients.

HERBAL TEAS

I'm a big fan of herbal teas, which I love for their soothing, healing, and revitalizing properties. There are three ways you can enjoy these fabulous natural concoctions. Of course you could grow your own. I'm lucky to have a back garden, where I grow some herbs myself—I use the leaves, flowers, roots, or even the whole plant, depending on how I feel— but a window box will do! If you can't be bothered with the business of growing, you can buy the dried leaves from a specialty herb store— or, to make things really easy, just buy herbal tea bags from a health food store or supermarket.

Try my list of favorite teas below, and as you get to know the different varieties and their health benefits, learn to listen to what your body is telling you. You'll soon sense which tea you need on any one particular day—the cleansing powers of dandelion, say, or the stress-busting qualities of linden flowers. You'll be amazed at the results!

NETTLE: MY NUMBER ONE FAVORITE

If there's one herbal tea you should reach for, this is it. All my clients know it's my staple favorite. It's loaded with minerals and iron, which makes it an excellent blood-builder—in fact, it's a tonic for the whole body. Personally, I always feel energized after drinking nettle tea, so I make sure I sit down to a cuppa a few times a week. Although nettle is not a laxative, it's such a great system cleanser that two to three cups a day can get your bowels going nicely. **NOTE TO MEN:** Nettle isn't just a woman's herb. Studies have shown that this plant may also help to prevent prostate problems.

DANDELION: THE LIVER CLEANSER

This herb is readily available. I've often gone out with my daughters and collected lovely yellow-flowered dandelions, which we then steep in hot water to make a delicious tea. That's how easy it can be. Dandelion is a fantastic liver cleanser, and can help to clear toxins from the body. It's also a diuretic, which means it can assist in getting rid of fluid retention and with weight loss. To make your own dandelion tea from fresh leaves, simply pour just boiled water over a small bunch of leaves, steep for 10 minutes, and then strain before drinking.

LINDEN FLOWER: THE STRESS-BUSTER

Linden flower tea can be effective in calming the nervous system and helping to induce sleep. If you suffer from that on-edge feeling, this is a good gentle tea for you.

MULLEIN: THE MUCUS-MOVER

If you have mucus or bronchial congestion, hayfever, earaches caused by excessive mucus, a hacking cough, or sinusitis, then start drinking this tea—fast!

PAU D'ARCO: THE YEAST-FIGHTER

Pau d'arco is a good antibacterial, antiviral, and antifungal. So, if you suffer from thrush, digestive problems, or general poor immunity, including frequent colds or flu, drink this tea. As soon as autumn ends, I load up on stocks of it for the winter!

FRESH MINT: A DIGESTIVE DYNAMO

Peppermint tea is refreshing, energizing, and soothing to the tummy. If you have a line down the middle of your tongue, which may suggest stomach weakness, then this should become your top tea.

   If you want the real thing, then buy a small mint plant from a supermarket or local garden center. Just clip off some fresh leaves, put them into a cup or pot of water, let it sit for a few minutes, and then drink. Bliss!

   The great thing about mint tea is that you can get it in restaurants, too— whether tea bags or fresh leaves.

SLIPPERY ELM: NATURE'S ANTI-INFLAMMATORY

This tea can soothe inflamed mucous membranes in the stomach, bowels, and urinary tract. Use it for diarrhea and ulcers, and for the treatment of colds, flu, and sore throats.

RED CLOVER: THE BLOOD-PURIFIER

Think of this tea as the antioxidant powerhouse. I sometimes use it for my clients on their detox days.

LEMON BALM: THE MOOD-LIFTER

Lemon balm has long been used as a mood-lifter and nerve-soother. It may also relieve tummy upsets and gas.

HAWTHORN: THE HEART-HELPER

A must-have for anyone who has a history of or family predisposition to heart ailments such as high blood pressure, hardening of the arteries, angina, high cholesterol, and varicose veins. Hawthorn has also been shown to improve circulation to the extremities.

OTHER GREAT HERBAL TEAS INCLUDE:

Bilberry
Chamomile
Elderflower
Fennel
Ginger
Green tea
Jasmine
Juniper berry
Lemongrass
Licorice
Passionflower
Raspberry leaf
Red clover
Sage
Spearmint

SPICES AND NATURAL FLAVORINGS

Spices and other natural flavorings have been used for centuries for their medicinal as well as their culinary qualities. Researchers are continuing to study the healing properties that can be offered by these natural remedies even today. They taste great, but don't go overboard with them—over-spicy food can irritate the lining of the stomach, so cut down on extra-hot curries and chiles and go for the gentler spices instead:

CARDAMOM (MEDIUM)

Cardamom contains essential oil properties and its main use is as a spice in coffees, curries, and other Asian and Middle Eastern foods. Available as pods and seeds, it has a pungent eucalyptus-like taste. Medicinally it is used as an aid to digestion. It is also thought to help colds, bronchitis, fevers, inflammatory conditions, and liver complaints.

CINNAMON (MILD)

Available in stick and powder form, cinnamon makes a great addition to desserts and Middle Eastern savory dishes. It is often used as an antidote to diarrhea and stomach upsets.

CUMIN (MILD)

Research has shown that cumin may stimulate the secretion of pancreatic enzymes, compounds necessary for proper digestion and nutrient assimilation. The seeds may also have anticarcinogenic properties. I use cumin, along with turmeric, in my Mung Bean Casserole (see page 183)—it gives real character to the dish. A great spice for detoxing.

FENNEL BULB (MILD)

The aniseed-y aroma of this bulb is one of my favorites. Delicious raw or cooked, it is an excellent source of fiber. It is also believed to be helpful in lowering elevated cholesterol levels as well as the diarrhea and constipation that are symptomatic of irritable bowel syndrome.

FENUGREEK (STRONG)

Fenugreek is one of the oldest known medicinal plants. Its dietary and medicinal uses date back to the ancient Egyptians, and today it is often used in Asian dishes. Fenugreek has always been valued for its health benefits—most commonly used to help manage diabetes and obesity.

GARLIC (STRONG)

Regular consumption of garlic can help lower high blood pressure and cholesterol levels. Its pungent flavor makes a delicious addition to virtually any savory dish, particularly pasta and stews.

GINGER (STRONG)

Ginger speeds metabolic rate. It's also a warming food that's perfect for veggie juices in the winter, good for colds and nausea, and is even said to help with mild depression. It happens to taste fantastic too.

HORSERADISH (STRONG)

Horseradish is a relative of the mustard family that acts as a digestive stimulant. Some people tell me it's great for clearing a blocked nose too!

NUTMEG (MILD)

Like other spices, nutmeg has aromatic, stimulant, and carminative properties. It has been used with advantage in mild cases of diarrhea, flatulent colic, and certain forms of dyspepsia. Good in sweet and savory dishes.

SAFFRON (MILD)

The dried stamens of a crocus flower, and said to be the most expensive spice in the world, saffron is used in many European and Asian dishes. It is believed to aid digestion, and relieves stomach upsets and tension.

TURMERIC (MILD)

Turmeric is an antioxidant that neutralizes free radicals and therefore may help to protect against cancer. It is also an anti-inflammatory and may help to protect the liver from a variety of toxins. Indian doctors have used turmeric to treat many ailments, from sprains to jaundice. I use it in my Mung Bean Casserole (see page 183).

VANILLA (MILD)

Vanilla is an aromatic stimulant that is thought to have aphrodisiac qualities. It's a wonderful spice for sweetening without sugar. Use the pod or extract.

IF YOU CAN'T TAKE THE HEAT

If hot spices don't agree with you, you'll know about it already. I definitely fall into that camp. I was in a restaurant once, on a romantic date, and asked for my meal to be served hot (as in warm temperature). About 10 seconds after eating it, I was overwhelmed by a terrible feeling of heat. Welts erupted all over my mouth, tears rolled down my cheeks, and I was burning up everywhere. It turned out they'd put lots of hot chiles in my dish, thinking I meant a different type of "hot."

MENU PLAN

Now you know my 10 Steps to Get It Together, here's an example of a typical menu plan I'd recommend to a client, along with a handy shopping list. It will take a while to get your pantry fully stocked, but simply add a few ingredients each week. You might want to use this plan to get started, or feel free to create your own and dive straight into the recipe section.

SATURDAY:
Shopping List
- Herbal teas: nettle, mint, chamomile
- Staples: mung beans, kidney beans, olive oil, wheat-free pasta, millet, brown rice
- Oils: olive
- Flavorings: vegetable bouillon powder (or ingredients for Vegetable Stock on page 229), miso soup packets, nutmeg, ginger, tamari sauce, bay leaves, turmeric, cumin
- Fruit: lemons, apples, mangoes, bananas, pineapple, blueberries, strawberries, pears
- Vegetables: onions, garlic, carrots, spinach, celery, black olives (pitted), pumpkin (or squash), asparagus, sweet potatoes, cabbage, green beans, avocados, cucumber, arugula (or watercress), lettuce, endive, radishes, red/yellow pepper, spring onions, bean sprouts, leeks, parsnips, marinated artichokes, cherry tomatoes, baby spinach, shiitake mushrooms
- Fresh herbs: parsley, cilantro, thyme, rosemary, basil
- Nuts: almonds, pine nuts, Brazil nuts, chestnuts
- Seeds: hemp, sunflower, pumpkin
- Milk: soy
- Protein: chicken breasts, salmon fillets, smoked tofu, goat cheese

SUNDAY EVENING:
- Make two batches of soup: Carrot and Almond (page 83) and Spinach (page 94). Transfer into airtight containers and keep in the fridge.

MONDAY
- On waking: Cup of warm water with a squeeze of fresh lemon juice
- Breakfast: Pineapple Prize Smoothie (page 61)
- Lunch: Carrot and Almond Soup (page 83), Green Salad (page 124)
- Dinner: Baked Salmon (page 146), add a small fillet for tomorrow's lunch
- Snacks: Whole pepper, pumpkin and sunflower seeds
- Drinks: 2 quarts still mineral water and various herbal teas or vegetable juices

TUESDAY
- On waking: Cup of warm water with a squeeze of fresh lemon juice
- Breakfast: Veggie Virgin Juice (page 52)
- Lunch: Carrot and Almond Soup (page 83), Baked Salmon (page 146) with lettuce
- Dinner: Lettuce and Cashew Wraps (page 143) with Gourmet Brown Rice (page 195), make extra filling for tomorrow's lunch
- Snacks: Toasted Nori Strips (page 213), berries
- Drinks: 2 quarts still mineral water and various herbal teas or vegetable juices

WEDNESDAY

▸ On waking: Cup of warm water with squeeze of fresh lemon juice
▸ Breakfast: Cinnamon Millet Porridge (page 76)
▸ Lunch: Spinach Soup (page 94), Lettuce and Cashew Wraps (page 143)
▸ Dinner: Baked Butterflied Chicken with Shiitake Mushrooms (page 139), make extra for tomorrow's lunch, and Crunchy Kale (page 202)
▸ Snacks: Small bowl blueberries, rice cakes with Guacamole Dip (page 208)
▸ Drinks: 2 quarts still mineral water and various herbal teas or vegetable juices

THURSDAY

▸ On waking: Cup of warm water with a squeeze of fresh lemon juice
▸ Breakfast: Fruit Salad (page 71)
▸ Lunch: Spinach Soup (page 94), Baked Butterflied Chicken with Shiitake Mushrooms (page 139)
▸ Dinner: Mung Bean Casserole (page 183), make extra and freeze
▸ Snacks: Brazil nuts, dates
▸ Drinks: 2 quarts still mineral water and various herbal teas or vegetable juices

FRIDAY

▸ On waking: Cup of warm water with a squeeze of fresh lemon juice
▸ Breakfast: Ginger Zinger (page 54)
▸ Lunch: Miso Soup (made from packet), Mung Bean Casserole (page 183)
▸ Dinner: Stuffed Zucchini (page 192)
▸ Snacks: Sunflower seeds, Black Olive Tapenade (page 208) with vegetable crudités
▸ Drinks: 2 quarts still mineral water and various herbal teas or vegetable juices

SATURDAY

▸ On waking: Cup of warm water with a squeeze of fresh lemon juice
▸ Breakfast: Mango Mania (page 61)
▸ Lunch: Best-Ever Beet Soup (page 86), Warm Chicken Salad (page 119)
▸ Dinner: Smoked Tofu and Bean Burger (page 155) with Sweet Potato Wedges (page 212) and Crunchy Kale (page 202)
▸ Snacks: Brazil nuts, grapes
▸ Drinks: 2 quarts still mineral water and various herbal teas or vegetable juices

SUNDAY

▸ On waking: Cup of warm water with a squeeze of fresh lemon juice
▸ Breakfast: Apple Action (page 66)
▸ Lunch: Chestnut Roast (page 153) served with lightly steamed cabbage
▸ Dinner: Hemp Pumpkin Soup (page 88)
▸ Snacks: Baked Apple (page 222), not right after lunch
▸ Drinks: 2 quarts still mineral water and various herbal teas or vegetable juices

EXTRA OPTIONS FOR VEGETARIANS

▸ The McKeith Shepherdess Pie (page 141)
▸ Mediterranean Black-Eyed Pea Casserole (page 145)
▸ Eggplant and Chickpea Tagine (page 162)
▸ Stir-Fried Vegetables with Arame (page 199)

CHAPTER 4

JUICES AND SMOOTHIES

JUICE JAMBOREE

Here's my biggest tip so far. Whenever you feel blue, toxic, unwell, or just plain tired, there's no better remedy than a glass of freshly made fruit or vegetable juices. It's a surefire way of injecting a cocktail of the most active health-giving compounds into your body.

But what's the point of waiting until you are falling apart before doing it? I'd like you to get into the habit of drinking three to four glasses of fresh juices a week (or at least on weekends) right now—before you get to the point of no return. Vegetable juices are even healthier than fruit, but whichever you go for, make sure you use organic produce. You will need a juicer for most of the juices in this chapter—if you have a food processor or blender but don't have a juicer yet, then feel free to start with the smoothie recipes (pages 60–66) and then progress to juices.

TO PEEL OR NOT TO PEEL?

When you buy organic, there's no need to ever peel, so think how much time you will save. I'm also a great advocate of leaving on the skin for its nutritional and energetic benefits—and this can apply even when the fruit and vegetables are juiced, so make sure you leave it on before putting them through the juicer. Whether you buy organic or non-organic, wash and scrub the skin thoroughly, and for non-organic fruit and vegetables, it is best to peel.

The juice recipes in this section are just some examples of what you can do. But be creative and try out as many combinations as you like. The sky's the limit!

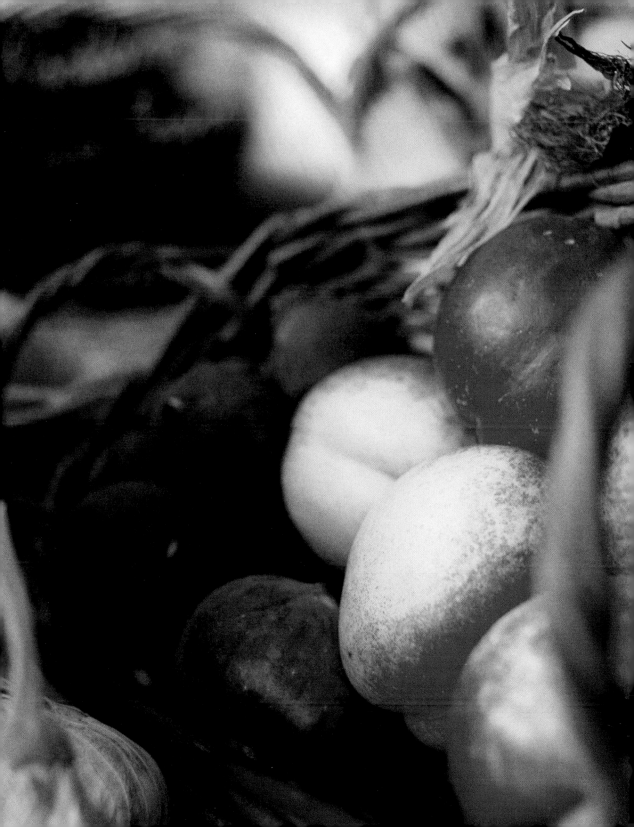

FRUIT JUICES

Most of you will already be used to the concept of juicing fresh fruits. Use the recipes below as a starting point, choosing familiar varieties at first, then go for more exotic choices when you're ready. For each recipe, just push the fruits through the juicer nozzle, then pour into a tall glass and serve.

PURE PEAR

A simple one this, just made from pears. Steep a few fresh mint leaves in it before drinking—it will add to the color and flavor, and will help your digestion!

SERVES 1–2
4 ripe pears, roughly chopped

CARIBBEAN COOLER

SERVES 1–2
Half a pineapple
1 papaya, seeded and roughly chopped

TOP TIP

Pineapple is a good source of vitamin C, which is great for your immune system and may help protect against colds.

BOUNTIFUL BERRIES

SERVES 1–2
1 pint strawberries, hulled
Half-pint raspberries
2 apples, roughly chopped

TOTAL CLEANSER

Another really easy one—you can either put the grapefruit through a juicer or use a citrus press.

SERVES 1–2
2 whole red grapefruits, roughly chopped or halved

WINTER WARMER

SERVES 1–2
4 apples, roughly chopped
Sprinkles of cinnamon to garnish

VEGETABLE JUICES

Vegetable juices are even healthier than fruit juices. They are my own particular preference, but they can be an acquired taste. It is a taste that can be enjoyed, however — it's simply a case of retraining your taste buds. After all, if we can enjoy the unnatural chemical flavors of soda and beer — which, frankly, don't taste that good initially — then we can certainly learn to love natural pure juices that come from the earth. When I was a student, I remember having friends who actually had to teach themselves how to like beer just to stay in with the crowd. The fact is that vegetable juices, once you're used to them, are delicious — and have side effects that can only be positive and beneficial to your health.

If you're new to vegetable juices and feel a bit apprehensive about drinking them, start off with this one:

VEGGIE VIRGIN JUICE FOR FIRST-TIMERS

Juice enough carrots to fill half an 8-ounce glass. Then fill the other half of the glass with fresh apple juice.

In other words, it's 50 percent carrots and 50 percent apple. Drink it for the first two weeks of your juice journey. After that, start to reduce the percentage of apple juice and either increase the amount of carrot or, preferably, add some juiced celery and juiced cucumbers. Before long, you'll find you're becoming a real vegetable juice junkie.

My aim is to get you to the stage where you are drinking vegetable juices without the apple or fruit juices mixed in. But don't fret over this. Just do your best until it feels right and feel free to experiment with all kinds of variations and creations of your own, always bearing in mind that adding carrot juice will make your veggie juices taste sweeter (and apple juice sweeter still). Even when you get used to drinking veggie juices on their own, you may find they make you feel nauseous if you drink them first thing in the morning. If you fall into this category, start off with fruit juices in the mornings, then continue with vegetable juices for the rest of the day.

VEGGIE VITALITY

This juice is so nutrient-dense that I regularly make it for my clients.
The recipe below is merely supposed to be a guideline—you may
have to experiment with the proportions to get the taste you want.
If you want more of a neutral taste, then add more cucumber;
if you want it sweeter, add more carrots or peppers.

SERVES 1–2
8 tomatoes, roughly chopped
7 carrots, trimmed
2 celery stalks, trimmed
Half a cucumber, halved lengthwise
1 handful cabbage leaves, roughly chopped
Half a yellow pepper, seeded and roughly chopped
2 green beans or snow peas
1 garlic clove, peeled
Half an onion, peeled

COOL AS A CUCUMBER

This is a great skin revitalizer! It's also one of the easiest juices
to make because cucumbers have a very high water content, which
makes them naturals for juicing.

SERVES 1–2
1 cucumber, halved lengthwise
2 celery stalks, trimmed
½-inch piece fresh ginger (optional)

You'll see that I've normally specified a ½-inch piece of ginger, but add as much as you like, according to taste.

SPROUT SURPRISE

SERVES 1–2
1 handful alfalfa sprouts
1 apple, roughly chopped
5 carrots, trimmed

GINGER ZINGER

This is a terrific breakfast juice that will perk up your whole system.

SERVES 1–2
2 apples, roughly chopped
2 ripe pears, roughly chopped
½-inch piece fresh ginger

WAKE-UP

SERVES 1–2
6 carrots, trimmed
1–2 apples, roughly chopped
½-inch piece fresh ginger

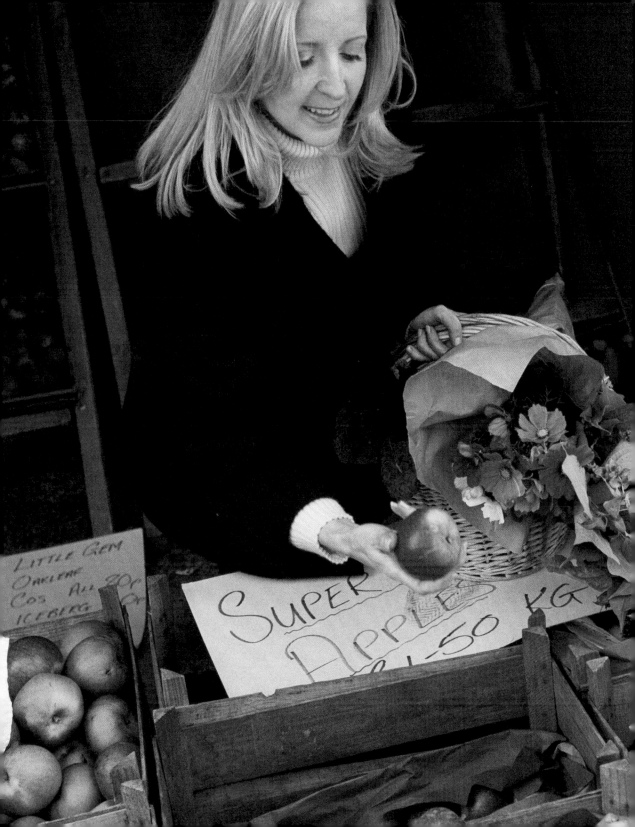

*Raw garlic in
a juice is fantastic
for helping to keep
blood pressure
in check.*

HAPPY TUMMY

This is a cool, refreshing stomach-easer. Adding the non-bitter aloe (available from a health food store) will really help soothe the gut and help digestion.

SERVES 1–2
2 apples, roughly chopped
1 lemon, skin and rind removed and halved
1 handful fresh mint
2 tbsp non-bitter aloe vera juice (optional)

ANTIBACTERIAL AND IMMUNITY BOOSTER

If you find this too sharp, add some celery or cucumber to neutralize the taste.

SERVES 1–2
1 handful broccoli sprouts, clover sprouts, or alfalfa sprouts
1 floret broccoli
1 small radish
2 carrots, trimmed
1 garlic clove, peeled, or 1 tsp chopped red onion

RELAXER

SERVES 1–2
1 cucumber, halved lengthwise
2 celery stalks, trimmed
3 lettuce leaves, roughly chopped

BEET BLISS FOR THE LIVER

Perfect for boosting flagging energy levels.

SERVES 1–2
3 carrots, trimmed
3 celery sticks, trimmed
Half a cucumber, halved lengthwise
1 small beet, roughly chopped

MINERAL MANIA

This juice can sometimes seem bitter on first tasting. The first few times you make it, feel free to add some apple juice to taste. For a real protein boost and even more minerals, add some liquid wild blue green algae.

SERVES 1–2
3 kale leaves, roughly chopped
2 fresh parsley sprigs
4 carrots, trimmed

FENNEL FUN

SERVES 1–2
Half a beet
4 carrots, trimmed
4 celery sticks, trimmed
1 fennel, quartered lengthwise

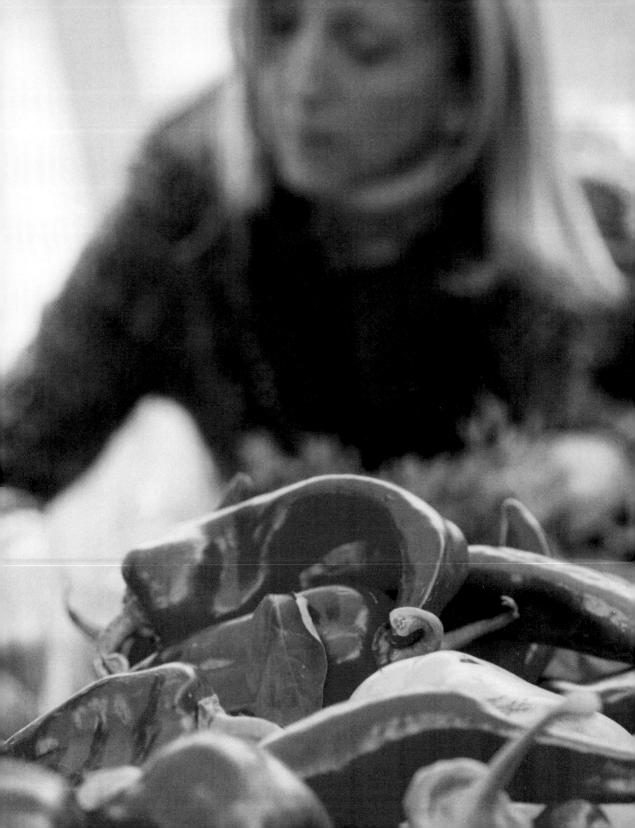

VEGGIE FACTS

- **Asparagus: Support for the kidneys**
  The alkaloid asparagine, found in asparagus (and also in potatoes and beets), stimulates the kidneys and has a strong diuretic effect.

- **Avocado (vegetable fruit): Heart protector** An excellent source of oleic acid, which is great for cardiovascular health. Also rich in vitamin E, which is essential for healthy skin.

- **Beans and snow peas: Protectors against diabetes** Pod vegetables are absorbed slowly and can help control insulin and reduce the risk of insulin resistance/diabetes.

- **Bean sprouts: Nutritional superstars**
  Bean sprouts are high in many minerals and vitamins that boost health and immunity.

- **Beets: Strength- and blood-builder**
  Very rich in immune-boosting beta-carotene and folate.

- **Broccoli: Cancer protection**
  Broccoli contains phytochemicals with significant anti-cancer effects.

- **Cabbage: Colon cancer protection**
  A rich vegetable source of vitamin C and a sulphur-containing compound called sinigrin that has excellent colon cancer fighting properties.

- **Carrot: Good for skin and eyes** Rich in beta-carotene, which is good for the immune system as well as for skin and eye health.

- **Celery: Cholesterol and blood pressure regulator** Celery contains active compounds called pthalides, which relax the muscles of the arteries that regulate blood pressure. It also has calming and diuretic properties.

- **Cress: Protector against cancer**
  Member of the brassica (cruciferous vegetable) family, with the same anti-cancer health benefits.

- **Cucumber: Heart protector**
  A strong diuretic, it can also help to lower blood pressure.

- **Dandelion leaves: Useful for arthritis**
  They help balance acid/alkaline levels in the body, which makes them useful in arthritic conditions.

- **Fennel: Irritable bowel syndrome relief** As a very good source of fiber, the fennel bulb may help to reduce elevated cholesterol levels as well as the diarrhea or constipation symptomatic of irritable bowel syndrome.

- **Onion: Immunity booster** Whether you have a cold or the flu, onions have amazing immune-boosting qualities. They are also antibacterial and antiseptic. (Leeks have similar but milder actions.)

- **Peppers: Immunity boosters** One of the richest sources of vitamin C, peppers provide support for the immune system. Yellow, red, and orange peppers also contain high levels of the antioxidant beta-carotene.

- **Tomato: Powerful antioxidant**
  A rich source of lycopene, which has strong antioxidant, anti-cancer, anti-aging properties.

- **Watercress: Good for bone health**
  An excellent source of magnesium and calcium for strong bones and hormonal balance. Watercress is also a good source of iron—to help beat fatigue—and sulphur, which is good for hair and nails.

SMOOTHIES

Blended fruit is a terrific energizer and cleanser and I love its taste and texture. In fact, I usually start my day with a fruit smoothie. When filming *You Are What You Eat*, I often have to leave home very early in the morning, so when I get up I have a cup of warm water and then make my smoothie. I make loads and put it all into tumbler containers which I take with me. You never know, you may well have seen me sitting on a train tucking into my nutrient-laden fruit delicacies.

I use my smoothies as a delivery medium for superfoods and added herbs. I think of them as vitamin infusions, or what I sometimes call my "nutrient shot." Here's my list of the key superfoods you can add to any of the smoothie recipes in this section.

KEY SUPERFOODS

- Barley grass powder
- Bee pollen granules
- Chlorella powder
- Gillian McKeith's Organic Energy Powder
- Flax seeds
- Liquid algae (the most easy-to-digest form of vegetable protein and a powerhouse of mineral nutrients)
- Non-bitter aloe liquid
- Spirulina powder
- Wheatgrass powder
- Wild blue green algae

All these superfoods should be available at your local health food store. Don't use all of them at once. Just pick one or two and use them in your smoothies for one particular day, week, or month and simply follow the instructions on the label for how much to use. When you've used the bottle(s) up, go out and get something else on the list. It's good to change your superfoods every now and again.

Smoothies are really easy to make. You can make them thick or thin, as you like—the thicker the smoothie, the more filling it will be. Practice makes perfect. Play around with all kinds of combinations and find out what you like.

If you want your smoothies to be less thick, then simply add some water.

MANGO MANIA

This is my number one top favorite smoothie. It's very filling and tastes heavenly—and it's a great way to get your bowels going.

SERVES 1–2
1 large mango, peeled, pitted, and roughly chopped
2 bananas, peeled and roughly chopped
Choice of superfood (see page 60)
1 handful each blueberries and raspberries, to serve

Blend the mango, banana, and choice of superfood until smooth and creamy. Put the blueberries and raspberries in a tall glass, reserving a few raspberries. Pour the smoothie over the berries and serve garnished with the reserved raspberries.

FOR A CHANGE...
Try Warmed Mango Mania, as a variation. Using the same ingredients as above, warm the mango and bananas in a pot with some water. Place the mixture in a blender, add your choice of superfood, and blend. Pour over the raw berries or some chopped apples. Perfect for the cold months, or if you need warming up!

PINEAPPLE PRIZE

SERVES 1–2
2 bananas, peeled and roughly chopped
1 mango, peeled, pitted, and roughly chopped
Half a pineapple, peeled and chopped

Blend until smooth and creamy. Add your favorite superfood for extra nutritional benefits!

BERRY BLASTER

SERVES 1–2
1 large or 2 small bananas, peeled and roughly chopped
1 handful blueberries, to serve

Blend the bananas until smooth and creamy. Put the blueberries in a tall glass. Pour the smoothie over the berries and serve.

VERY BERRY BLAST-OFF

SERVES 1–2
2 handfuls strawberries, hulled
2 handfuls raspberries
2 apples, cored and roughly chopped
½ cup non-bitter aloe or water (to blend the apple).
1 tsp liquid algae
1 handful blueberries, to serve

Blend the berries, apples, and liquid algae until smooth and creamy. Put the blueberries in a tall glass. Pour the smoothie over the berries and serve.

SEXY STARTER

SERVES 1–2
1 handful strawberries, hulled
1 handful blueberrries
1 handful raspberries
1 large banana, peeled and roughly chopped

Blend until smooth and creamy, then serve.

PEACH MEDLEY

SERVES 1–2
4 peaches, pitted and quartered
2 ripe pears, cored and roughly chopped
1 apple, cored and roughly chopped

Add ½ cup water. Blend until smooth and creamy, then serve.

MINERAL MOVER

SERVES 1–2
3 ripe pears, cored and roughly chopped
2 apples, cored and roughly chopped
(slightly warmed so they will blend easily)
3 apricots, pitted
1 tsp liquid algae

Blend until smooth and creamy, then serve.

BERRY BEAUTY

SERVES 1–2
2 handfuls strawberries, hulled
1 large or 2 small mangoes, peeled, pitted, and roughly chopped

Blend until smooth and creamy, then serve.

VITAMIN C COCKTAIL

You haven't lived till you've tasted this one!

SERVES 1–2
1 pineapple, peeled and roughly chopped
2 handfuls strawberries, hulled
1 handful gooseberries, blueberries, or raspberries, to serve

Blend the pineapple chunks and strawberries until smooth and creamy. Put your choice of berries in a tall glass. Pour the smoothie over the berries and serve.

PEAR PERFECTION

SERVES 1–2
6 ripe pears, cored and roughly chopped
2 bananas, peeled and roughly chopped

Blend until smooth and creamy, then serve. Add a little water if the mixture is too thick.

KIWI COOLER

SERVES 1
2 kiwis
1 apple or pear, cored and roughly chopped

Blend until smooth and creamy, then serve. Add a little water if the mixture is too thick.

PINEAPPLE PUREE

SERVES 1–2
1 pineapple, peeled and roughly chopped
2 small bananas, peeled and roughly chopped
1 peach, pitted and chopped, to serve

Blend the pineapple and bananas until smooth and creamy. Put the chopped peach in a tall glass. Pour the smoothie over the peach and serve.

FRUIT FRENZY

SERVES 1–2
3 peaches, pitted and quartered
3 ripe pears, cored and roughly chopped
3 plums, pitted
1 handful raspberries, blackberries, or other berries of your choice, to serve

Blend the peaches, pears, and plums until smooth and creamy. Put the berries in a tall glass. Pour the smoothie over the berries and serve.

YUM-YUM DELIGHT

Kids can make smoothies too. This one was invented by my wee daughter. I love it—and so do my clients.

SERVES 1–2
2 plums, pitted
2 nectarines, pitted and quartered
2 ripe pears, cored and roughly chopped
Half a handful blueberries
12 strawberries, hulled

Add ½ cup water. Blend until smooth and creamy, then serve.

APPLE ACTION

Another kids' invention—inspired by my other (even wee-er) daughter.

SERVES 1–2
2 apples, cored and roughly chopped
3 ripe pears, cored and roughly chopped
1 handful strawberries, hulled and chopped (optional)

Add ½ cup water. Blend until smooth and creamy. Garnish with chopped-up strawberries if desired.

JUICY SMOOTHIE

This is a fantastic, filling juice-smoothie combination—great for detox days! It's absolutely delicious—and full of essential "thinny" fats.

SERVES 1–2
6 carrots, trimmed
1 apple, cored and roughly chopped
1 ripe avocado, peeled, pitted, and roughly chopped
10 basil leaves
1 lemon wedge

Push the carrots and apple through a juicer. Blend the juice with the avocado and basil leaves. Squeeze a dash of lemon into the smoothie and serve.

PEAR AND STRAWBERRY SMOOTHIE

SERVES 1–2
2 ripe pears, cored and roughly chopped
½ pound strawberries, hulled

Blend until smooth and creamy, then serve.

FRUIT FACTS

- Apple: Cholesterol-buster Their pectin content may lower cholesterol.
- Apricot: Sight-saver Their vitamin A content promotes good vision.
- Banana: Great destressor Rich in the mineral potassium, they're fantastic for destressing and lowering high blood pressure.
- Blueberry: The sexy superfruit A good source of zinc and other antioxidants and nutrients associated with sex hormones in men and women.
- Cantaloupe: Lung-saver Beta-carotene and vitamin C content in cantaloupe could be life-savers if you're exposed to secondhand smoking.
- Cherry: Nature's joint rescuer Cherries may help a wide range of conditions affecting the joints, including arthritis, gout, and rheumatism.
- Cranberry: Good for urinary tract infections Their unique antibacterial action helps to maintain urinary tract health.
- Date: Blood-builder Dates are high in potassium and dietary fiber. They are also a good source of energy-boosting iron.
- Fig: Bone-strengthener Figs are a fruit source of calcium, a mineral that has many functions, including promoting bone density.
- Grapefruit: Antibacterial detoxer Phytochemicals and antioxidants in grapefruit help fight disease and infection.
- Grape: Blood-purifier Grapes contain ingredients that may help to purify your glands and blood.
- Kiwi: Heart-helper Kiwi is an excellent source of nutrients that protect the blood vessels and heart.
- Lemon and lime: Good blood building Their high vitamin C content helps iron absorption. They're great gas-busters too.
- Mango: Immune booster Vitamin C powerhouses with impressive levels of disease-fighting carotenoids, vitamin A, folate, potassium, and fiber.
- Papaya: Colon-helper The nutrients and fiber in papaya have been shown to be helpful in the prevention of colon cancer.
- Peach: Nature's anti-cold remedy A good source of vitamin C, which is vital for the proper function of a healthy immune system.
- Pear: Age-fighter A great source of vitamin C and copper—both antioxidant nutrients that help protect cells in the body from oxygen-related damage caused by free radicals.
- Pineapple: Energy-booster An excellent source of manganese, thiamin, and riboflavin, which are important for energy production.
- Plum: Digestive aid Rich in bromelain, a sulphur-containing group of enzymes that can aid the digestion of proteins.
- Prune: Appetite-suppressant The soluble fiber in prunes promotes a sense of satisfied fullness after eating by slowing down the rate at which food leaves the stomach. So prunes can also help prevent overeating and weight gain.
- Raisin: Bone-builder A top source of boron—a mineral that is critical for bone health and the prevention of osteoporosis (bone softening).
- Raspberry: Brain food Antioxidant phytonutrients in raspberries can help improve learning capacity and motor skills.
- Strawberry: Anti-cancer compounds The ellagitannin content of strawberries has been associated with helping to prevent cancer.
- Watermelon: Anti-inflammatory They contain nutrients that can help quench the inflammation that contributes to conditions such as asthma, diabetes, colon cancer, and arthritis.

CHAPTER **5** BREAKFASTS

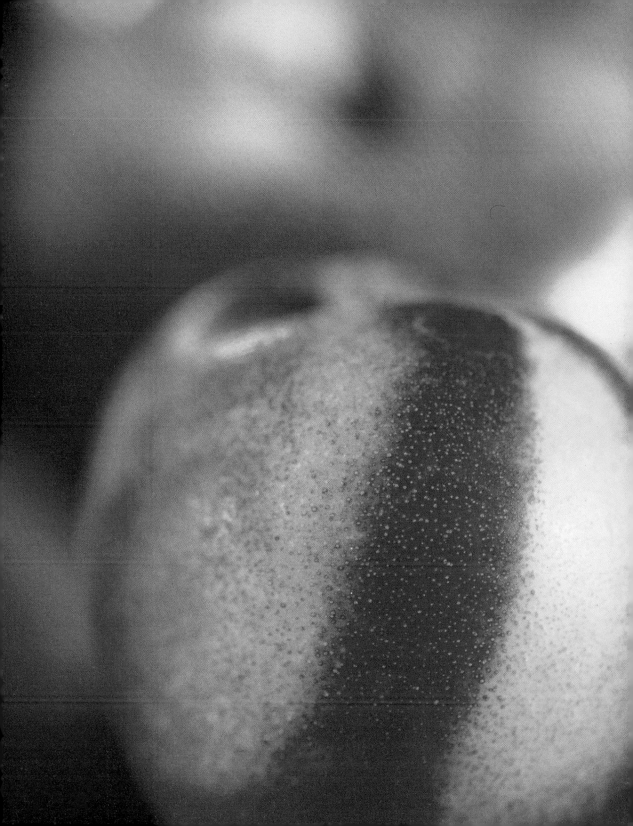

I ALWAYS SAY THAT YOU SHOULD BREAKFAST LIKE A KING. WHEN YOU WAKE UP IN THE MORNING, YOU HAVE IN EFFECT BEEN FASTING FOR SEVERAL HOURS. THE BODY IS IN NEED OF FOOD, AND DIGESTIVE ENERGY IS AT ITS STRONGEST. WHEN YOU EAT A PROPER BREAKFAST, IT IS LIKE GIVING YOURSELF AN ENERGY INJECTION, AND THERE ARE NOW STRONG, CREDIBLE STUDIES WHICH SHOW THE BENEFITS OF EATING A HEALTHY BREAKFAST: INCLUDING WEIGHT LOSS, ENHANCING MEMORY, AND IMPROVING BRAIN FUNCTION.

PERSONALLY, I USED TO FIND THAT IF I EVER MISSED BREAKFAST I WOULD SUFFER FROM HEADACHES AND MID-MORNING ENERGY SLUMPS. NOW MY FAVORITE WAY TO START THE DAY IS EITHER WITH A SMOOTHIE (PAGES 60–66) OR PORRIDGE (PAGES 75–77). YOU CAN EVEN HAVE SOUP FOR BREAKFAST (PAGE 74), AND ON THE WEEKENDS YOU MIGHT WANT TO INDULGE IN A FRITTATA (PAGE 78) OR HOMEMADE BEANS ON TOAST (PAGE 79).

FRUIT SIMPLING

This simply means eating one single fruit for maximum ease of digestion. Remember to wash all fruit. Your raw fruit of choice might be any one of the following:

SERVES 1

½ **whole pineapple**

1 whole papaya

1 whole mango

2 whole apples

A bunch of grapes, red or white

A bowl of blueberries, strawberries, or raspberries

AUTUMN FRUIT SALAD

SERVES 4 / KEEPS FOR TWO DAYS IN THE FRIDGE

4 apples, quartered, cored, and chopped

4 ripe pears, quartered, cored, and sliced

8 plums, halved, pitted, and sliced

1 cup freshly pressed apple juice

Combine the ingredients and serve immediately.

FRUIT SALAD WITH WARM PEAR SAUCE

SERVES 4 / KEEPS FOR TWO DAYS IN THE FRIDGE

4 ripe pears, cored and chopped

2 tbsp lemon juice

½ **pound strawberries, hulled**

½ **pound raspberries**

½ **pound blueberries**

1. Place the pears in a small saucepan with the lemon juice. Add enough water to cover. Bring to a boil, reduce the heat, and cook gently over low heat until quite soft. Remove from the liquid and allow to cool. Blend in a food processor or with a handheld blender until smooth. Add a little water if you prefer the sauce to be thinner.
2. Mix the berries together in a bowl and pour over the pear sauce. Serve immediately or chill until ready to serve.

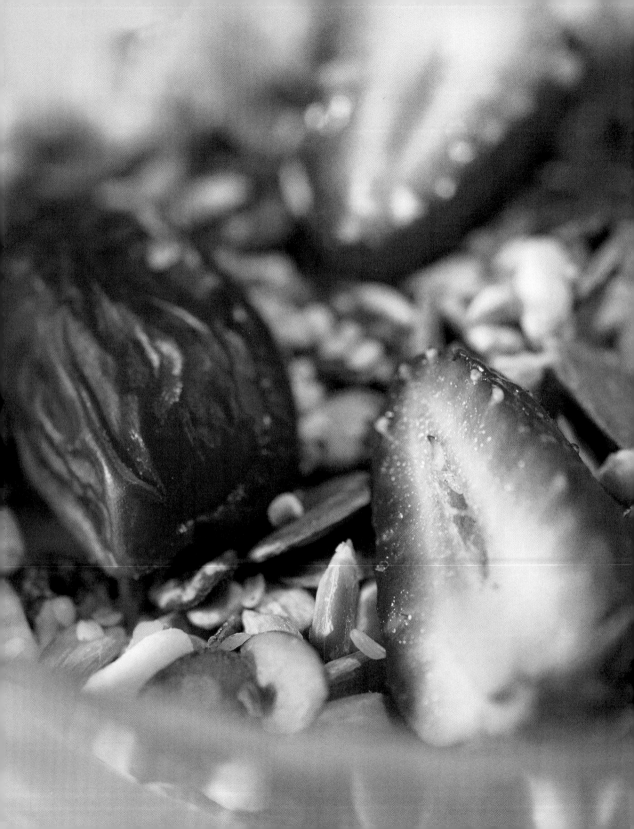

MUESLI

The key when developing your own muesli recipe is not to mix too many different ingredients. Keep it simple. See below for ingredient ideas. If you are food combining, then don't include any fruit in your muesli (see page 16).

GRAIN
Barley flakes
Buckwheat
Millet flakes
Oat bran
Puffed corn
Puffed millet
Puffed rice
Rice bran
Rice flakes
Rolled barley
Rolled oats
Rolled rice
Rolled rye
Rolled wheat
Soy grits
Wheat bran
Wheat germ

FRUIT
Apples
Apricots
Bananas
Blackberries
Blueberries
Currants
Dates
Dried papaya
Figs
Kiwis
Peaches
Pears
Plums
Prunes
Raisins
Raspberries
Strawberries

SEEDS
Alfalfa seeds
Flax seeds
Hemp seeds (shelled)
Poppy seeds
Sesame seeds
Sunflower seeds

NUTS
Almonds
Brazil nuts
Cashews
Coconut
Hazelnuts
Macadamias
Peanuts (unsalted)
Walnuts

OTHER
Apple juice (freshly pressed)
Barley malt syrup
Cinnamon
Rice milk
Soy milk
Spelt milk

MISO BARLEY SOUP

SERVES 1
¼ cup pearl barley, soaked for 12 hours or overnight in cold water
1 packet instant miso soup

1. Drain the barley.
2. Bring ½ cup water to a boil, add the barley, and bring
back to a boil. Lower the heat and simmer for 10–15 minutes.
3. Add the packet of soup. Stir and serve.

BREAKFAST SOUP BLITZ

This is one that I make all the time because it's so quick and easy.

SERVES 1–2
¼ cup shiro miso
2 packets white miso
2 red onions, peeled and diced
Half a leek, washed, trimmed, and thinly sliced
Half a 16-ounce block tofu, diced
Half a fennel bulb, trimmed and thinly sliced
½ pound curly kale, roughly chopped

1. Bring 1 cup water to a boil. Add the shiro miso and
white miso, lower the heat, and simmer for 2 minutes.
2. Add all the other ingredients, stir, then turn off the heat
and allow to stand for 8 minutes before serving.

NOTE ABOUT HOT CEREAL

*The simplest hot cereal to make is oatmeal with soy, millet, amaranth, spelt, or rice milk.
Simply combine 1 cup rolled oats with 2 cups grain milk in a pan, bring to a boil, then
lower the heat and simmer for 15–20 minutes. Oats are a great source of fiber and complex
carbohydrates, good for sustained energy. A diet high in natural fiber and low in processed
foods can also be beneficial for heart health.*

QUINOA PORRIDGE

Quinoa comes in two forms: flakes and grain. I like the texture and flavor of the grain best — it takes a little bit longer to cook, though we are only talking a matter of minutes. See what you like best, so try both. And of course, the flakes are super-quick if you are in a rush. Soy or rice milk may be used as an alternative to the apple juice for a creamier texture.

SERVES 2–4
1½ cups quinoa grains
Quarter of a cinnamon stick
½ cup freshly pressed apple juice

1. Place the quinoa, cinnamon, apple juice, and 3¾ cups water in a medium saucepan. Bring to a boil, then lower the heat and simmer for 7–10 minutes, or until the grains are translucent.
2. Turn off the heat and allow to stand for 15 minutes before serving. Delicious!

VANILLA BARLEY PORRIDGE

SERVES 2–4
1½ cups barley groats, soaked in water overnight
Half a vanilla pod
2 tsp flax seeds

1. Drain the barley.
2. Place the barley in a medium to large saucepan along with the vanilla pod and 3¾ cups water. Bring to a boil, then lower the heat and simmer for 15 minutes.
3. Serve warm, sprinkled with flax seeds.

CINNAMON MILLET PORRIDGE

SERVES 2–4
1½ cups millet
1 cinnamon stick
Zest of half a lemon
2 tbsp shelled hemp seeds

1. Place the millet, cinnamon, and lemon zest, together with
3¾ cups water in a medium pan and bring to a boil.
Lower the heat and simmer for 1 hour.
2. Serve warm with the hemp seeds sprinkled on top.

BUCKWHEAT, LEMON, AND GINGER PORRIDGE

SERVES 2–4
1½ cups buckwheat groats
Juice and zest of 1 lemon
1-inch piece fresh ginger, peeled and grated
1 pinch dried mixed herbs
1 handful shelled hemp seeds

1. Place the buckwheat, lemon juice and zest, ginger, herbs, and 3¾ cups water in a medium pan. Bring to a boil, then lower the heat and simmer for 20 minutes.
2. Top with the hemp seeds and serve immediately.

BRAN PORRIDGE

Hemp seeds contain the most perfect ratio of omega-3, omega-6, and omega-9, the good essential fatty acids for energy, glowing skin, lustrous hair, and balanced hormones. And they taste great too.

SERVES 2–4
1½ cups mixed oat bran, oat groats, and rolled oats
2 tbsp shelled hemp seeds
2 tsp agave syrup (optional)

1. Place the grains and 3¾ cups water (or rice milk for extra flavor) in a medium saucepan. Bring to a boil, then lower the heat and simmer, stirring regularly, until thickened.
2. Turn off the heat and allow to stand for a few minutes. Before serving, sprinkle some hemp seeds on top and drizzle over the agave syrup, if using.

FRITTATA WITH CHERRY TOMATOES AND BABY SPINACH

I do not advocate the overeating of eggs but as a special treat try this recipe now and again.

SERVES 2–3

6 organic eggs

1 tsp olive oil

½ pound cherry tomatoes, Cut in half

¾ pound baby spinach

Chopped fresh basil

Chopped fresh parsley

1. Preheat the oven to 400°F.
2. Whisk the eggs with 2 tablespoons of water.
3. Heat the oil in a cast-iron pan or frittata plate with 1 tablespoon of water. Add the tomatoes and spinach and cook until the spinach begins to wilt. Sprinkle over the herbs.
4. Pour in the eggs and transfer to the preheated oven.
5. Bake for 10–12 minutes, until well-risen and golden brown.
6. Slice in wedges and serve with a side salad.

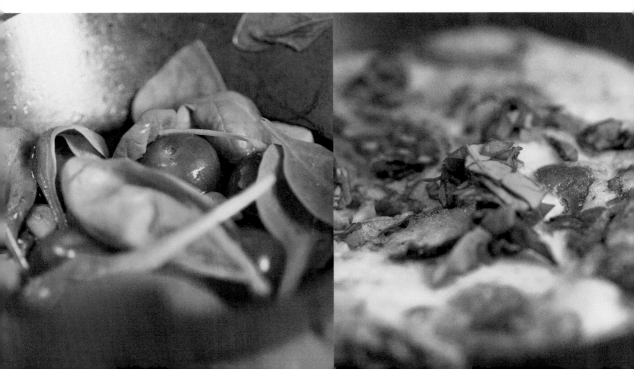

GRILLED PEACHES

SERVES 4
4 ripe peaches, halved and pitted
½ pound strawberries, hulled and halved
½ pound blueberries

1. Preheat the broiler on its highest setting.
2. Place the peaches cut side up on the broiler pan.
3. Cook for 3–4 minutes, or until lightly browned.
4. Transfer to 4 plates, top with the fresh berries, and serve.

HOMEMADE BEANS
ON SQUASH BREAD TOAST

SERVES 4
14-ounce can organic tomatoes
16-ounce can navy beans
4 slices Gluten-Free Squash Bread (see page 212)
1 tsp chopped fresh oregano

1. Place the tomatoes in a small pan and bring to a boil.
Lower the heat and simmer for 20 minutes, breaking up the
tomatoes as they cook. Add the beans and cook for an additional
5 minutes.
2. Toast the bread, top with the bean mixture, and serve
garnished with the fresh oregano.

CHAPTER 6

SOUPS

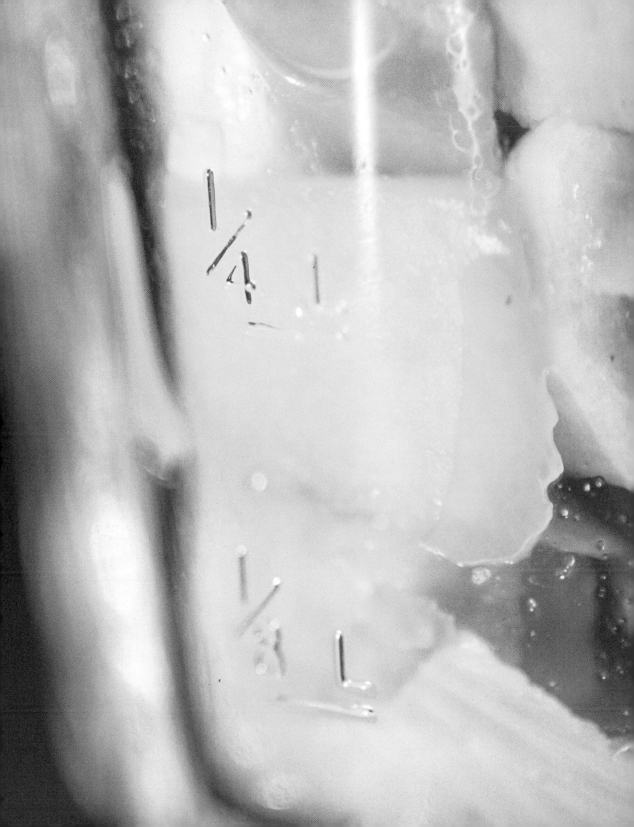

YOU'LL FIND EACH SOUP IN THIS CHAPTER FANTASTIC FOR YOU IN DIFFERENT WAYS. TRY ALL THE RECIPES OUT, BUT ALSO THINK ABOUT USING THEM AS A GUIDE TO CREATING VARIATIONS THAT YOU LIKE. BE ADVENTUROUS WITH FLAVORINGS— ADDING HERBS AT THE END OF COOKING CAN MAKE A HUGE DIFFERENCE. DON'T BE SHY—THROW IN HANDFULS OR BUNCHES, RATHER THAN A LEAF HERE AND THERE. HERBS CAN CHANGE EVERYTHING IF YOU LET THEM MAKE A STATEMENT!

GET CREATIVE WITH SEEDS TOO. USE HEMP, FLAX, AMARANTH, OR POPPY SEEDS. THEY'RE NOT ONLY DELICIOUS AND FLAVORFUL, BUT PACKED WITH MINERALS AND ESSENTIAL FATTY ACIDS THAT ARE CRUCIAL FOR WEIGHT MANAGEMENT, ENERGY, AND OPTIMUM DIGESTION.

FOR EXTRA FLAVOR I ALWAYS RECOMMEND THAT YOU USE ROASTED VEGETABLE STOCK (SEE PAGE 230) OR VEGETABLE STOCK (SEE PAGE 229) AS AN ALTERNATIVE TO BOUILLON POWDER OR STOCK CUBES. MAKE LOADS OF STOCK IN ADVANCE AND FREEZE IT. THAT WAY YOU'LL ALWAYS HAVE SOME ON HAND WHEN YOU DECIDE SOUP IS ON THE MENU THAT DAY!

CARROT AND ALMOND SOUP

Carrots are a source of anti-aging antioxidants, while almonds are a powerhouse of nutrients, incuding magnesium, which is important for supporting adrenal function. Low levels of magnesium have been associated with nervous tension, so almonds are a natural stress-buster.

SERVES 4
2 onions, peeled and chopped
2 garlic cloves, peeled and chopped
6 carrots, trimmed, peeled, and sliced
2 celery stalks, trimmed and chopped
1 tbsp wheat-free vegetable bouillon powder
1 cup ground almonds
2–3 tbsp chopped fresh cilantro, stalks reserved
2–3 tbsp chopped fresh parsley, stalks reserved

1. Place the onions, garlic, carrots, and celery in a large saucepan. Add 6¼ cups boiling water and the bouillon powder. Bring to a boil and add the herbs.
2. Lower the heat and simmer for 20 minutes, or until vegetables are tender when pierced with a knife.
3. Remove from the heat and allow to cool slightly. Strain, reserving the stock. Blend the vegetables in a food processor or with a handheld blender until smooth.
4. Return the mixture to the pan and add the ground almonds and enough of the reserved stock to make a soup-like consistency.
5. Reheat, then divide among warmed soup bowls and serve garnished with chopped fresh cilantro and parsley.

FOR A CHANGE ...
This soup is also very good made with sweet potatoes. Just add one sweet potato, peeled and diced, in place of two of the carrots and cook as above.

CREAMY BROCCOLI SOUP

Broccoli is a friend to your liver. It contains a compound called sulphorophane, which has been shown to inhibit the growth of free radicals, those nasty molecules that age us and make us feel tired.

SERVES 4
1 fennel bulb, trimmed and diced
1 wheat-free vegetable stock cube
3 whole heads broccoli, cut into florets and stems thinly sliced
1 handful fresh tarragon
1 handful fresh sage
1 pint alfafa sprouts (or any other sprouted seeds of choice)

1. Bring a medium pan of water to a boil, then add the fennel and stock cube. Lower the heat and simmer for 5–7 minutes. Add the broccoli, including the stems, and simmer for an additional 4–5 minutes.
2. Remove from the heat and add the tarragon and sage. Allow to cool, then blend the soup in a food processor or with a handheld blender until smooth.
3. Divide among warmed soup bowls. Sprinkle with the sprouts and serve immediately.

TURNIP AND LEEK SOUP

A firm favorite in our house. Leeks belong to the same family of vegetable as onions and garlic and contain many of the same beneficial nutrients. They are also a good source of manganese, vitamin B_6, vitamin C, folate, and iron. This combination makes leeks helpful in stabilizing blood sugar, helping to slow the absorption of sugars from the intestinal tract and ensure that they are properly metabolized in the body.

SERVES 4
1 turnip, trimmed, peeled, and diced
1 wheat-free vegetable stock cube
1 tbsp wheat-free vegetable bouillon powder
6 celery stalks, trimmed and roughly chopped
6 leeks, washed, trimmed, and chopped
3 small onions, peeled and chopped
¼ cup chopped fresh tarragon

1. Place 3 cups water in a large saucepan, bring to a boil, and add the turnip, stock cube, and bouillon powder. Lower the heat and simmer for 10 minutes.
2. Add the celery, leeks, and onions and simmer for an additional 15 minutes.
3. Remove from the heat and allow to cool, add the tarragon, then blend in a food processor or with a handheld blender to your desired consistency.
4. Reheat, divide among warmed soup bowls, and serve.

BEST-EVER BEET SOUP

If you are tired, this is the soup for you. Go to a mirror, pull down your lower eyelid, and check to see the color of your inner inside lid. If it's pale, you may need more iron. And of course, you need my best-ever soup.

SERVES 4
1 tbsp olive oil
1 onion, peeled and chopped
1 garlic clove, peeled and chopped
2 celery stalks, trimmed and sliced
1 large parsnip, trimmed, peeled, and grated
6 small raw beets, trimmed, peeled, and grated
1 wheat-free vegetable stock cube
1 tsp wheat-free vegetable bouillon powder
1 tbsp cider vinegar
1 sweet potato, peeled and diced
Third of a cucumber, peeled and diced
2 tbsp finely chopped fresh dill

1. Place the oil, onion, garlic, and celery in a large saucepan with 3 tablespoons of water. Cook over medium-low heat, stirring frequently, for 3–4 minutes, until soft but not colored.
2. Add the parsnip, beets, stock cube, and bouillon powder to the pan with 4¼ cups cold water. Bring to a boil, then lower the heat and simmer for 30 minutes.
3. Stir in the vinegar and sweet potato and continue to simmer for 10 minutes, or until the vegetables are tender when pierced with a knife.
4. Ladle into warmed soup bowls and serve garnished with the diced cucumber mixed with the dill.

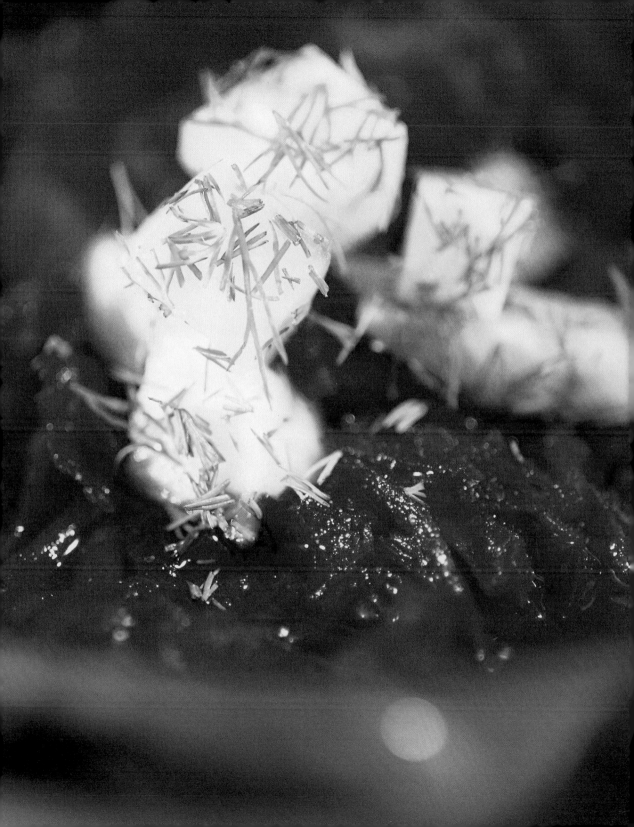

HEMP PUMPKIN SOUP

Pumpkin has a delicious sweet flavor. It helps
to regulate sugar balance and is high in potassium
and vitamin C, and its seeds contain zinc—a libido-
and immune-system booster. Hemp seeds provide
a perfect ratio of essential fatty acids, more so
than any other seed.

SERVES 4
1 pumpkin or seasonal squash, peeled,
seeded, and cut into 1-inch pieces
1 bunch asparagus, roughly chopped
(tips reserved for a salad)
2 large sweet potatoes, peeled and
cut into 1-inch pieces
3 carrots, trimmed, peeled, and chopped
6 onions, peeled and roughly chopped
1 wheat-free vegetable stock cube
1 garlic clove, peeled and chopped
2 tbsp chopped fresh cilantro
2 tbsp shelled hemp seeds
2 tbsp pumpkin seeds

1. Bring a large pan with 1 quart water to a boil, then
add the pumpkin or squash, asparagus, sweet potatoes,
carrots, onions, and stock cube. Bring back to a boil,
then lower the heat and simmer for 10–15 minutes, or
until the vegetables are tender when pierced with a knife.
2. Remove from the heat and add the garlic and cilantro.
3. Allow to cool and then blend in a food processor or
with a handheld blender to your desired consistency.
4. Reheat gently. Divide among warmed bowls and
serve garnished with the seeds.

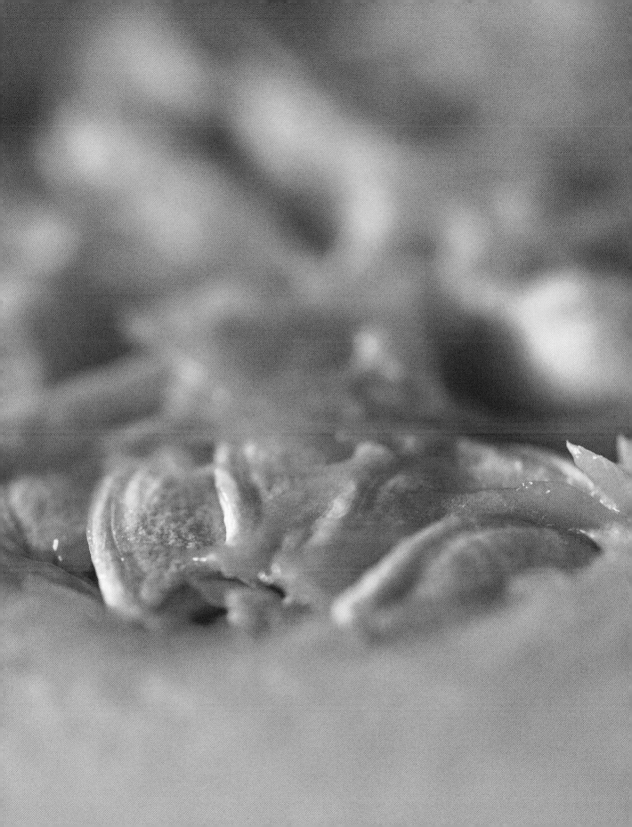

WHITE BEAN AND CABBAGE SOUP

SERVES 4
1 onion, peeled and thinly sliced
2 celery stalks, trimmed and thinly sliced
1 whole white cabbage, cut in half, cored, and thinly sliced
1 wheat-free vegetable stock cube
1 tbsp wheat-free vegetable bouillon powder
15-ounce can lima beans, drained and rinsed
2 tbsp chopped fresh parsley
¼ cup fresh garden peas

1. Place the onion, celery, cabbage, stock cube, and bouillon powder in a medium pan with enough water to cover.
2. Bring to a boil, then lower the heat and simmer for 30–40 minutes, adding a little more water if necessary.
3. Add the lima beans and simmer for an additional 10 minutes.
4. Divide among warmed soup bowls and serve immediately, garnished with the parsley and peas.

BUTTERNUT SQUASH AND
SWEET POTATO SOUP

The digestive dynamo of all soups. If you have a line down the middle
of your tongue or teeth marks round the sides—it could be a sign of
a weakened spleen and tummy—then this soup is for you. It will help
you absorb more nutrients from all the foods you eat.

SERVES 4

1 butternut squash, peeled, seeded,
and diced
1 sweet potato, peeled and diced
2 carrots, trimmed, peeled, and sliced
1 fennel bulb, trimmed and chopped
6 shallots, peeled and thinly sliced
1 wheat-free vegetable stock cube

1 garlic clove, peeled and chopped
¼ cup chopped fresh parsley
1 bunch radishes, trimmed
and chopped
4–6 tbsp pumpkin seeds (optional)

1. Bring a large pan half-filled with water to a boil. Add the squash,
sweet potato, carrots, fennel, shallots, and stock cube.

2. Bring to a boil, then lower the heat and simmer for 10–12 minutes.

3. Remove from the heat and add the garlic.

4. Allow to cool, then strain the vegetables into a large bowl to keep
the stock.

5. Add half the stock to the vegetables and blend in a food processor
or with a handheld blender to desired consistency.

6. Reheat the soup gently, adding more of the reserved stock if necessary.

7. Divide among warmed soup bowls and serve garnished with the parsley,
radishes, and pumpkin seeds, if using.

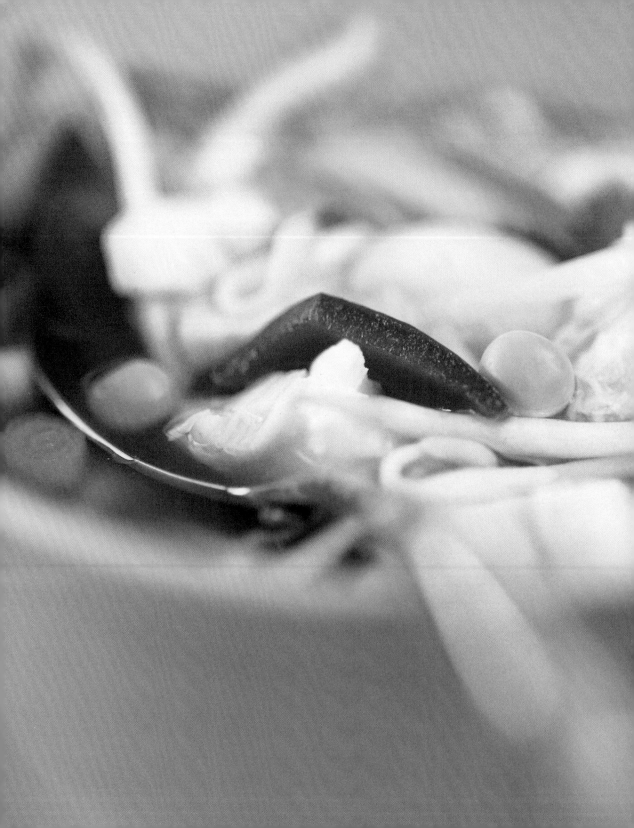

TEN-MINUTE MISO FISH SOUP

This soup has been a true success with my TV participants because it is so easy to make and can be ready in 10 minutes. It is loaded with nutrients and miso is a tremendous source of good bacteria.

SERVES 4
1 garlic clove, peeled and thinly sliced
1-inch piece fresh ginger, peeled and thinly sliced
1 packet instant miso soup
¼ pound skinless boned white fish, cut into chunks
8 snowpeas, trimmed and sliced
1 red pepper, seeded and chopped
1 bunch bok choy, thinly sliced
2 spring onions, trimmed and sliced
1 handful bean sprouts
1 handful fresh garden peas

1. Bring 2 cups water to a boil in a medium pan. Add the garlic, ginger, and miso soup. Boil for 1 minute and then add the fish, snap peas, and red pepper. Bring back to a boil and skim any foam that accumulates from the top with a slotted spoon. Cook for 2 minutes.

2. Add the bok choy and spring onions and cook for an additional minute.

3. Divide among warmed soup bowls. Add the bean sprouts and peas and serve immediately.

SPINACH SOUP

If you are late in from work and are really starving, here is a soup you can whip up in just a few minutes. Spinach contains good levels of vitamin B_6, which helps lower levels of homocysteine in the body. High levels of homocysteine are associated with an increased risk of heart attack or stroke.

SERVES 4
1 onion, peeled and finely chopped
1 tsp olive oil
1 pound fresh spinach
1 wheat-free vegetable stock cube
1 handful parsley stalks
Fresh nutmeg, to taste
1 cup soy milk (optional)
1 tbsp pumpkin seeds
1 handful fresh baby spinach leaves

1. Place the onion, olive oil, and 1 tablespoon of water in a large pan. Cook over medium-low heat for 2–3 minutes, until soft.
2. Add the spinach, 2 cups boiling water, the stock cube, and parsley stalks and cook for 5–7 minutes. Allow to cool slightly, remove the parsley, then blend in a food processor or with a handheld blender until smooth.
3. Return to the pan, season with a little nutmeg, stir in the soy milk (or 1 cup water or Vegetable Stock on page 229) and reheat gently.
4. Divide among warmed soup bowls and serve garnished with the pumpkin seeds and baby spinach leaves.

SUPER GREEN KALE SOUP

If you feel tired, irritable, constipated, or crave sweet things, then this is
a great soup for you. Getting your fair share of dark green leafy vegetables
is extremely important. Kale is an excellent source of vitamin C — just one
cup contains nearly 90 percent of the recommended daily intake. It also
contains magnesium, which has been shown to help migraine sufferers.

SERVES 4
1 tbsp olive oil
1 large onion, peeled and sliced
1 garlic clove, peeled and crushed
2 turnips, trimmed, peeled, and chopped
2 wheat-free vegetable stock cubes
2 zucchinis, trimmed and sliced into ½-inch pieces
½ pound curly kale, rinsed and drained
1 handful chopped fresh dill

1. Heat the oil in a large saucepan and gently cook the onion and garlic
over medium-low heat for 4–5 minutes, stirring constantly so the onion does
not brown. Add the turnips and cook for an additional 3 minutes.
2. Add 3¼ cups boiling water and the stock cubes. Bring to a boil, then lower
the heat and simmer for 10 minutes.
3. Add the zucchini and kale and simmer for an additional 5 minutes.
4. Allow to cool, then blend in a food processor or with a handheld blender
until smooth.
5. Divide among warmed soup bowls and serve garnished with dill.

RAW AVOCADO AND CUCUMBER SOUP

Including as much raw food as possible in your food regime is essential.
Avocado contains minerals, including iron and potassium, and it also contains
the all-important essential fatty acids. It's high on my list as
a source of good fats.

SERVES 4
3 cucumbers, peeled
1 large ripe avocado, pitted, peeled, and roughly chopped
Juice of 1 lemon
1 garlic clove, peeled and chopped
3 tbsp chopped fresh mint leaves
1 red pepper, seeded and finely chopped
1 yellow pepper, seeded and finely chopped
1 tbsp thinly sliced fresh chives and chervil

Optional:
Pine nuts
Celery or sea salt

1. With an electric juicer, process two of the cucumbers into juice and reserve.
2. Roughly chop the remaining cucumber and blend with the avocado, lemon
juice, garlic, and mint in a food processor or with a handheld blender until
smooth. Add the reserved cucumber juice and blend again until mixed through.
3. Chill until ready to serve. Divide among cold soup bowls and serve garnished
with the peppers, chives, and chervil.
4. Options for those new to the raw soup: You can opt for a pinch of celery or
sea salt. Top with pine nuts, too, for extra flavor.

TUSCAN BEAN SOUP

SERVES 4

2 onions, peeled and roughly chopped

2 tsp olive oil

2 celery stalks, trimmed and chopped

1 leek, washed, trimmed, and finely chopped

6 garlic cloves, peeled and chopped

1 tsp dried oregano

1 tbsp chopped fresh basil

16-ounce can organic tomatoes

1 tbsp fresh chopped parsley

16-ounce can no-salt mixed
beans, drained and rinsed

For the salsa:

1 tsbp chopped yellow pepper

1 tbsp chopped green pepper

1 tbsp chopped red onion

1. Place the onions in a medium saucepan with the olive oil
and 1 tablespoon of water and cook for 2–3 minutes. Add the celery
and leek and cook for an additional 3–4 minutes.

2. Add the garlic and oregano, cook for 2 minutes, then add the basil
and tomatoes and cook for an additional 5 minutes.

3. Add 1 cup boiling water and the chopped parsley and cook for
5 more minutes, then add the beans.

4. To make the salsa, mix the peppers and onions together in a small bowl.

5. Divide the soup among warmed bowls and serve garnished with the pepper
salsa.

SLEEPY LETTUCE SOUP

When I tell people to try lettuce soup, they look at me as if I've gone mad. It can taste delicious, I promise you, and has great health benefits. Lettuce has diuretic qualities and is therefore great for weight loss. It also helps dry up damp in the body—in other words, if you suffer from edema, swollen ankles, or yeasty problems such as thrush, lettuce is for you. Best of all, it contains a compound which is relaxing to the nervous system. So instead of counting sheep, try my Sleepy Lettuce Soup.

SERVES 4
1 tbsp olive oil
1 large onion, peeled and chopped
1 garlic clove, peeled and crushed
1 pound, potatoes, peeled and cut into 1-inch cubes
2 tsp wheat-free vegetable bouillon powder
½ cup millet
1 large head romaine lettuce, washed and roughly shredded
4 tbsp cup chopped fresh chervil or parsley

1. Heat the oil with a little water in a large saucepan. Add the onion and garlic and cook for 3–4 minutes, stirring occasionally.
2. Add the potatoes and cook for 2 additional minutes.
3. Add 4¼ cups water, together with the bouillon powder and millet. Bring to a boil, then lower the heat and simmer for 15 minutes, or until the vegetables are tender when pierced with a knife.
4. Add the lettuce and cook for 2–3 minutes, or until just wilted.
5. Allow to cool before blending in a food processor or with a handheld blender until smooth along with 2 tablespoons of the fresh chervil or parsley.
6. Return to the pan to reheat, adding a little water if necessary.
7. Divide among warmed soup bowls and serve garnished with the remaining fresh chervil or parsley.

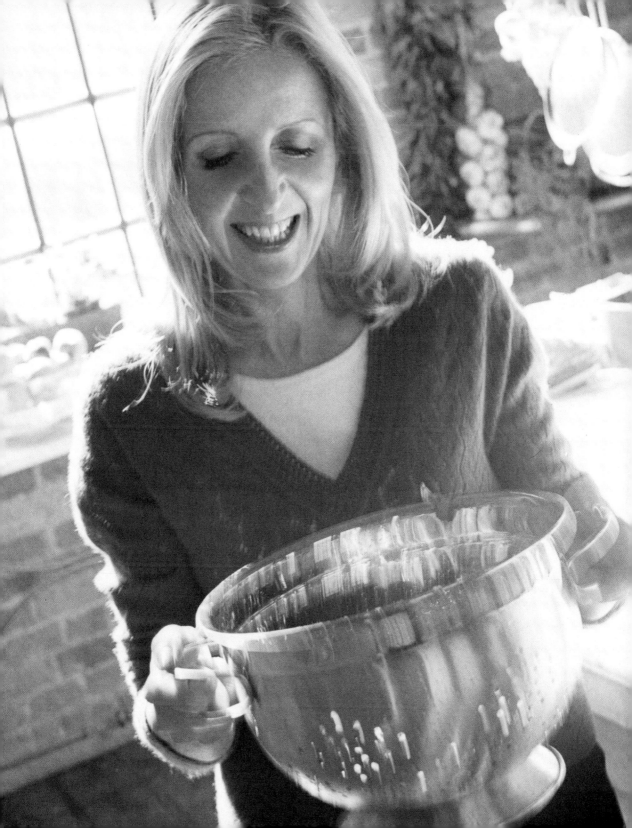

ZUCCHINI AND ASPARAGUS SOUP

This soup is perfect for using up any leftover asparagus trimmings. Asparagus contains inulin, which can promote the growth and activity of intestine-friendly bacteria.

SERVES 4
1 onion, peeled and finely chopped
1 pound zucchini, trimmed and cut into large pieces
1 bunch asparagus trimmings
1 quart Roasted Vegetable Stock (see page 230)
1 handful fresh rosemary leaves
Pumpkin seed oil or hemp oil

1. Place the onion with 1 tablespoon of water in a large pan and cook for 2–3 minutes. Add the zucchini, asparagus, and vegetable stock. Bring to a boil, then lower the heat and simmer for 10 minutes.
2. Allow to cool, then blend in a food processor or with a handheld blender along with the fresh rosemary until smooth.
3. Divide among warmed soup bowls, drizzle over a little pumpkin seed or hemp oil, and serve.

FENNEL AND HAZELNUT SOUP

Fennel contains a powerful combination of phytonutrients, including anethole, which may enhance immune response. It is also an excellent source of vitamin C. Hazelnuts are rich in healthy fats.

SERVES 4
1 small onion, peeled and thinly sliced
3 fennel bulbs, trimmed, thinly sliced, and cored
1 quart Roasted Vegetable Stock (see page 230)
1 handful parsley
¼ pound chopped hazelnuts (raw and unsalted)
Soy milk

1. Place the onion with 1 tablespoon of water in a large pan and cook for 2–3 minutes. Add the fennel and vegetable stock. Bring to a boil, then lower the heat and simmer for 20 minutes.
2. Allow to cool slightly, then blend in a food processor or with a handheld blender until completely smooth. Add the nuts and parsley and process for an addtional 30 seconds.
3. Return to the pan, adding a little soy milk to achieve a creamy consistency. Divide among warmed soup bowls and serve.

WARMING SPLIT PEA SOUP

This is my kids' favorite soup—they just can't get enough of it. Its ingredients help to strengthen digestion and the spleen, your energy battery. Great for cold winter days.

SERVES 4
½ pound yellow split peas, soaked for 12 hours or overnight in cold water
1 wheat-free vegetable stock cube
1 tsp wheat-free vegetable bouillon powder
1 onion, peeled and sliced
1 sweet potato, peeled and chopped
3 carrots, trimmed, peeled, and thickly sliced
4 sprigs fresh mint
4 handfuls fresh baby spinach leaves

1. Place the soaked peas in a sieve and rinse well in cold water. Transfer to a large saucepan and cover with 6⅓ cups cold water, the stock cube, and the bouillon powder. Bring to a boil, then lower the heat and simmer for 25 minutes. Remove any foam that rises to the surface with a spoon.
2. Add all the other vegetables and simmer for an additional 15–20 minutes, or until the vegetables are tender when pierced with a knife.
3. Remove from the heat and allow to cool, then blend the soup in a food processor or with a handheld blender until smooth.
4. Return to the pan and reheat, stirring gently. Divide among warmed soup bowls and garnish with the fresh mint. Add the spinach leaves before serving.

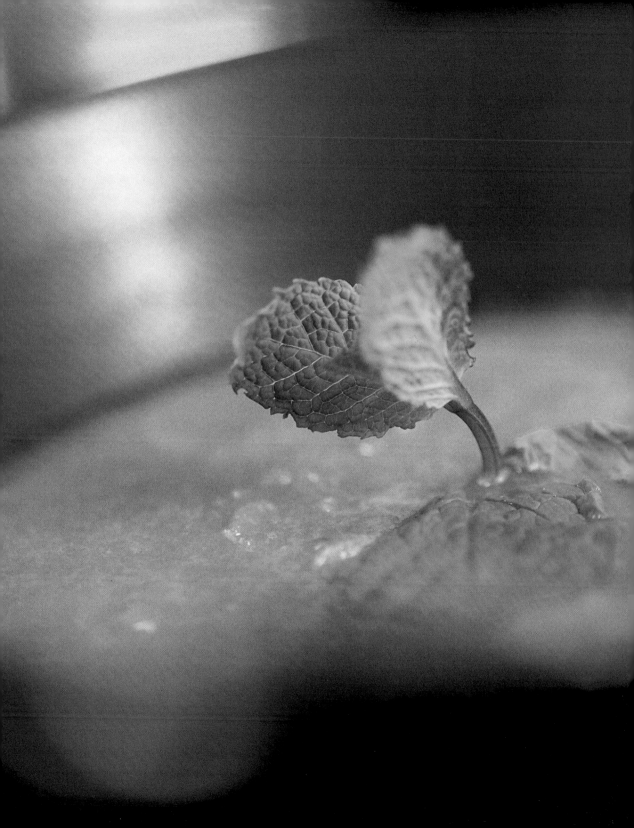

VELVETY CAULIFLOWER SOUP

SERVES 6
2 tbsp olive oil
2 garlic cloves, peeled and crushed
2 onions, peeled and chopped
3 leeks, washed, trimmed, and sliced
Half a celeriac, scrubbed, trimmed, and chopped
1 head cauliflower, trimmed and cut into small florets
1 tsp ground cumin (optional)
3 tbsp chopped fresh parsley

1. Heat the oil in a large saucepan or flameproof casserole with
1 tablespoon of water over low heat.
2. Add the garlic, onions, leeks, and celeriac and cook very gently
for 20 minutes, or until softened, stirring occasionally .
3. Add the cauliflower florets, 4 cups cold water, and the cumin, if using.
Bring to a boil, then reduce the heat and simmer for 10–15 minutes, stirring
occasionally, until the cauliflower is tender when pierced with a knife.
4. Leave to cool for 5 minutes, then blend in a food processor or with
a handheld blender until smooth. Return to the pan and reheat gently.
If necessary, add more water (or Vegetable Stock, see page 229).
5. Serve in warmed bowls and garnish with the chopped fresh parsley.

TOMATO AND HERB SOUP
WITH PEARL BARLEY

Tomatoes are rich in the antioxidant lycopene. Low levels of lycopene are associated with a higher risk of prostate cancer.

SERVES 4
1½ cups pearl barley
2 pounds ripe tomatoes, chopped
1 onion, peeled and finely chopped
1 garlic clove, peeled and chopped
1 pinch grated fresh mace
1 handful fresh basil leaves and stalks
1 tsp chopped fresh oregano

1. Soak the pearl barley in cold water for 10 minutes. Drain and rinse well.
2. Place the tomatoes, onion, garlic, and mace in a large pan and cook over low heat for 20 minutes. Break up the tomatoes with a spoon as they cook.
3. Add 2 cups boiling water and the basil stalks. Simmer for 10 minutes, then remove from the heat and allow to cool.
4. Pass the mixture through a food mill or roughly blend in a food processor or with a handheld blender. Return to the pan and add the barley. Bring back to a boil, then lower the heat and simmer for 20 minutes. Add more water if needed.
5. Divide among warm bowls and serve garnished with basil leaves and oregano.

CHAPTER 7

SALADS AND LUNCH-BOXES

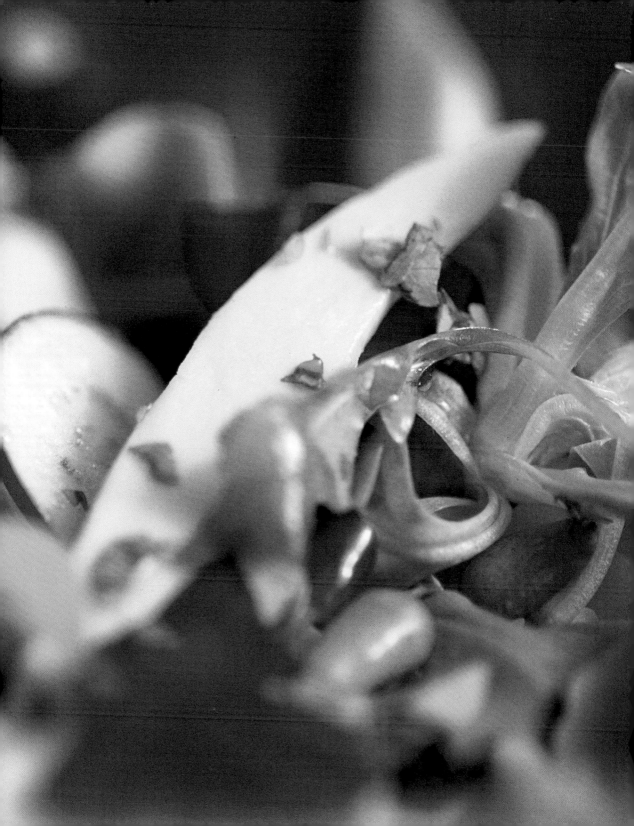

I HIGHLY RECOMMEND AT LEAST ONE SALAD A DAY FOR EXTRA VITALITY. THEY ARE PERFECT FOR LUNCH AND ADD THAT EXTRA, RAW ZIP TO A COOKED MEAL. I REMEMBER FILMING WITH A FAMILY FOR THE TV PROGRAM *YOU ARE WHAT YOU EAT* AND BEING FACED WITH THE CHALLENGE THAT THEY ALL HATED SALAD, PARTICULARLY THE EIGHT-YEAR-OLD SON. LUCKILY, WHEN I PRESENTED HIM WITH A CRUNCHY ALTERNATIVE TO LIMP LETTUCE LEAVES—BEAN SPROUTS, YELLOW PEPPERS, BROCCOLI FLORETS, CABBAGE SHREDS, BEET SHREDS, RADISHES, AND CHICORY WITH A FENNEL AND TOMATO DRESSING—HE COULD NOT GET ENOUGH. "I'VE NEVER HAD ANYTHING TASTE SO GOOD AS THIS," HE SAID!

YOU CAN THROW A TASTY SALAD TOGETHER IN JUST A FEW MINUTES. MY FAVORITE IS A CRUNCHY VEGGIE SALAD. IF YOU ARE IN A RUSH, SIMPLY RUSTLE UP SOME SNOW PEAS, PEAS IN A POD, BROCCOLI FLORETS, AND FENNEL WITH A SQUEEZE OF LEMON. THIS TASTES GREAT WITH MY HEARTY LENTIL STEW (SEE PAGE 167). BE ADVENTUROUS. AS YOU'LL SEE, THERE'S MUCH MORE TO SALADS THAN LETTUCE, CUCUMBER, AND TOMATO . . .

AVOCADO AND BARLEY SALAD WITH PUMPKIN SEEDS

A fantastic way to get a good supply of those fat-burning essential fatty acids and the ever-important sexy mineral zinc.

SERVES 4
2 ripe avocados
1 cup cooked barley
¼ pound snow peas or snap peas, trimmed
2 spring onions, trimmed and finely chopped
1 small bunch radishes, trimmed and sliced
1 tbsp chopped fresh parsley
1 tbsp pumpkin seeds
⅓ pound mixed salad leaves
Dressing:
2 tsp pumpkin seed oil
1 tsp freshly squeezed lemon juice

1. Peel, pit, and slice the avocados and mix with the barley, snow peas, or snap peas, spring onions, radishes, parsley, and pumpkin seeds.
2. Divide the salad leaves among salad plates and pile the avocado mixture on top.
3. Add 1 tablespoon of water to the salad dressing ingredients, mix together well, and spoon a little dressing over each salad. Serve immediately.

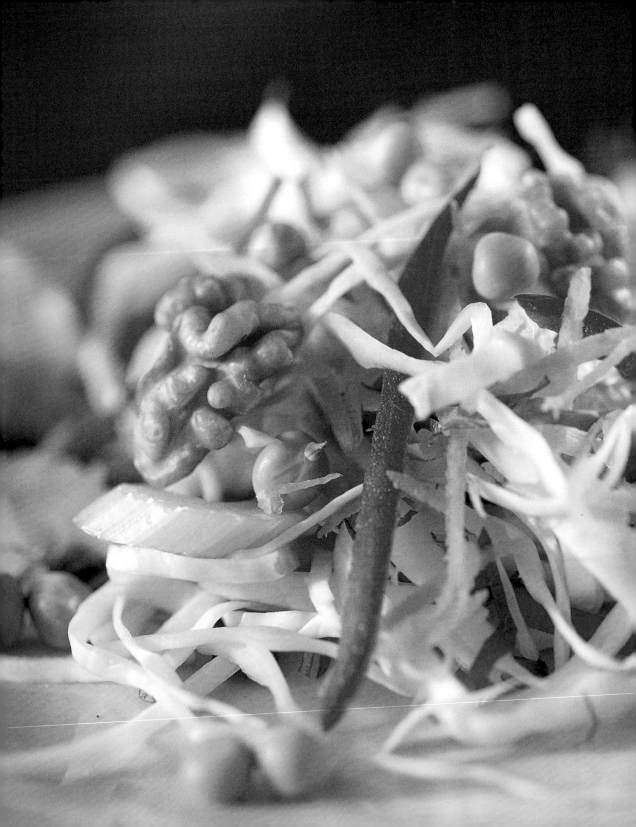

CRUNCHY WALNUT COLESLAW

This is a treat for your body. Cabbage contains compounds that help your liver to process toxins more effectively and walnuts have been found to help lower levels of bad cholesterol. Kohlrabi looks like a little turnip. It can be eaten raw in salads as here, used in soups, or baked. So eat my crunchy coleslaw at least once a week.

Serves 4
Quarter of a white cabbage, cored and finely shredded
Quarter of a kohlrabi, peeled and grated (optional)
4 carrots, trimmed, peeled, and grated
2 celery stalks trimmed and thinly sliced
1 red pepper, seeded and thinly sliced
2 ounces fresh garden peas
3 spring onions, trimmed and thinly sliced
1 cup walnut halves
1 tbsp chopped fresh parsley
Dressing:
3 tbsp olive oil
1 tbsp cider vinegar
1 tsp Dijon mustard
1 garlic clove, peeled and crushed

1. Combine all the vegetables for the coleslaw in a large bowl.
2. Using a food processor or handheld blender, blend the dressing ingredients together with 3 tablespoons of water until creamy.
3. Pour the dressing over the salad and toss to combine.
4. Divide the salad among salad plates and serve garnished with the walnuts and parsley.

NAVY BEAN SALAD

This salad is full of fiber and a rich source of vitamin B, essential for weight management and the nervous system. Cider vinegar is excellent for digestion.

SERVES 4

½ pound fresh navy beans, soaked for 12 hours or overnight in cold water

1 onion, peeled and finely chopped

1 tsp miso paste

1 wheat-free vegetable stock cube

1 celery stalk, trimmed and thinly sliced

3 tbsp chopped pickles

Half a red pepper, seeded and thinly sliced

Half a yellow pepper, seeded and thinly sliced

¼ pound sauerkraut

¼ pound mixed baby lettuce leaves

2 tbsp sunflower seeds

¼ cup chopped fresh parsley

Dressing:

1 tbsp olive oil

1 tsp cider vinegar

1. Bring 1 quart of water to a boil in a large pan and add the beans, onion, miso, and stock cube. Bring back to a boil, then lower the heat and simmer for 20–30 minutes, until the beans are soft but not breaking up. Drain.

2. Add 1 tablespoon of water to the dressing ingredients, mix well, and toss into the beans.

3. Mix the celery, pickles, peppers, and sauerkraut together and arrange with the salad leaves on a large platter.

4. Scatter the beans over the salad and serve garnished with the sunflower seeds and parsley.

SPRING SALAD

I use the Chinese root daikon in this salad. I have found it to be helpful for congestion. Asparagus is often used to help with PMS-related water retension.

SERVES 4
¼ pound snap peas
1 bunch asparagus, trimmed and cut into bite-size pieces
1 carrot, trimmed, peeled, and cut into thin julienne (matchstick) strips
Quarter of a daikon, peeled and cut into large julienne (matchstick) strips

1 bunch radishes, trimmed and cut into quarters
½ cup pumpkin seeds
1 tablespoon shelled hemp seeds
Dressing:
1 tsp umeboshi paste
2 tbsp rice vinegar
2 tsp olive oil

1. Bring a large pot of water to a boil and blanch the vegetables one at a time, starting with the snap peas and asparagus, which need to be cooked for 2–3 minutes, then the carrot for 3–4 minutes, and finally the daikon for 4–5 minutes. Remove each vegetable as it is cooked with a slotted spoon and refresh under cold water. Drain well.

2. Add 1 tablespoon of water to the dressing ingredients and mix well.

3. In a large salad bowl, mix the cooked vegetables with the radishes. Spoon over the dressing and serve garnished with the pumpkin and hemp seeds.

TABBOULEH

I use buckwheat groats in my tabbouleh as they are gluten-free,
so easy on the digestive tract. I also use lots of parsley—it's one
of the most important herbs for providing vitamins to your body
and is also an excellent digestive restorative.

SERVES 4
1 cup buckwheat groats
6 tbsp chopped fresh mint
¾ cup steak chopped fresh parsley
1 large beefsteak tomato, halved, seeded, and finely chopped
1 cucumber, peeled, seeded, and diced
2 onions, peeled and finely chopped
1 tbsp olive oil
Juice of 1 lemon
1 pinch of dried mixed herbs
Lettuce leaves
4 lemon wedges

1. Rinse and drain the buckwheat groats. Bring a medium pan of
water to a boil, add the buckwheat groats and cook for 10 minutes
or until tender. Drain and allow to cool.
2. Mix the mint, parsley, tomato, cucumber, onion, olive oil, lemon
juice, and dried mixed herbs together in a large bowl. Mix through
the buckwheat groats and chill until ready to serve.
3. Pile high on a serving platter and serve garnished with lettuce
and lemon wedges.

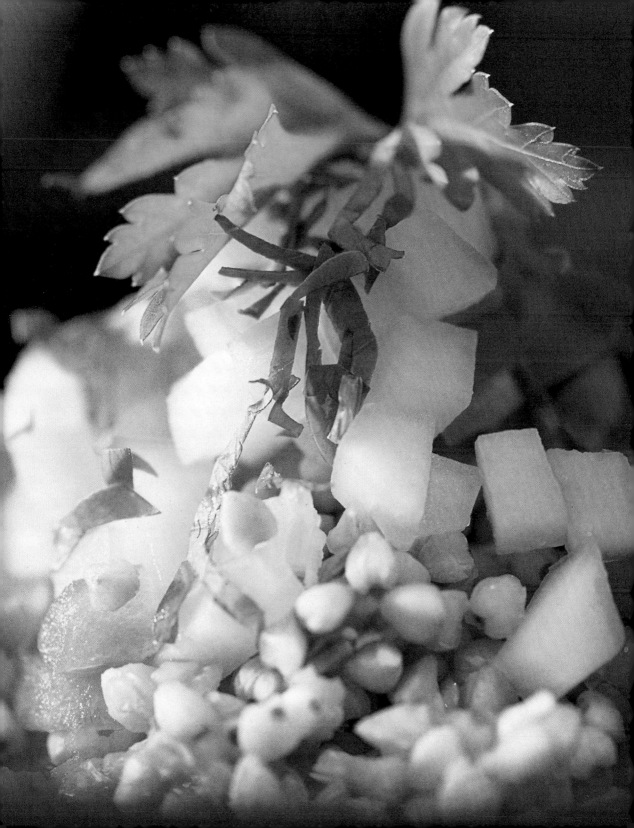

SEA VEGETABLE AND SPROUT SALAD

The idea of eating seaweed in a salad may seem wacky at first. The reality is that sea vegetables can offer a wonderful complement to many meals, both in taste and nutrition. Wakame is sweet in flavor and a good source of calcium.

SERVES 4

2 strips wakame sea vegetable
Half a cucumber, peeled and cut into julienne (matchstick) strips
1 pint cherry tomatoes, halved
1 baby Boston lettuce, leaves separated
4 ounces canned corn, drained and rinsed
½ pound mung bean sprouts

Dressing:
1 tsp soy or tamari sauce
1 tbsp olive oil
1 tbsp grated orange rind
1 tsp grated fresh ginger
2 tbsp freshly pressed apple juice

1. Rinse the wakame under cold water for 1 minute, then soak in a bowl of cold water for 2–3 minutes.
2. Place the dressing ingredients in a small bowl, add 3 tablespoons of water, and whisk well to combine.
3. Drain the wakame and chop into bite-size pieces. Place in a small bowl with half the dressing and leave to marinate.
4. Arrange the remaining ingredients in a large salad bowl, add the wakame and the rest of the dressing, toss the salad, and serve immediately.

WARM VEGETABLE QUINOA SALAD

Quinoa is a supergrain and contains all the essential amino acids
as well as being a rich source of calcium.

SERVES 4

1 red pepper, seeded and halved

1 yellow pepper, seeded and halved

1 zucchini, trimmed and thinly sliced

1 small red onion, peeled and thinly sliced

½ cup quinoa grains

4 sprigs fresh thyme

2 sprigs fresh rosemary

2 tbsp pine nuts

¼ pound fresh arugula

3 tbsp chopped fresh basil

4 lemon wedges

1. Preheat the oven to 400°F.

2. Place the peppers cut side up on an ovenproof baking dish and
scatter the zucchini and red onion over the top. Place in the oven
and roast for 15 minutes.

3. Meanwhile, rinse and drain the quinoa and add to a medium pan
of boiling water, along with the thyme and rosemary. Cook for
8–10 minutes. Drain and set aside.

4. Scatter 1 tablespoon of the pine nuts over the peppers and cook
for an additional 5–10 minutes.

5. Remove the baking dish from the oven and spoon the quinoa
into the pepper halves.

6. Scatter with the arugula, fresh basil, and the remaining pine nuts and
arrange the lemon wedges (for squeezing) on top. Serve immediately.

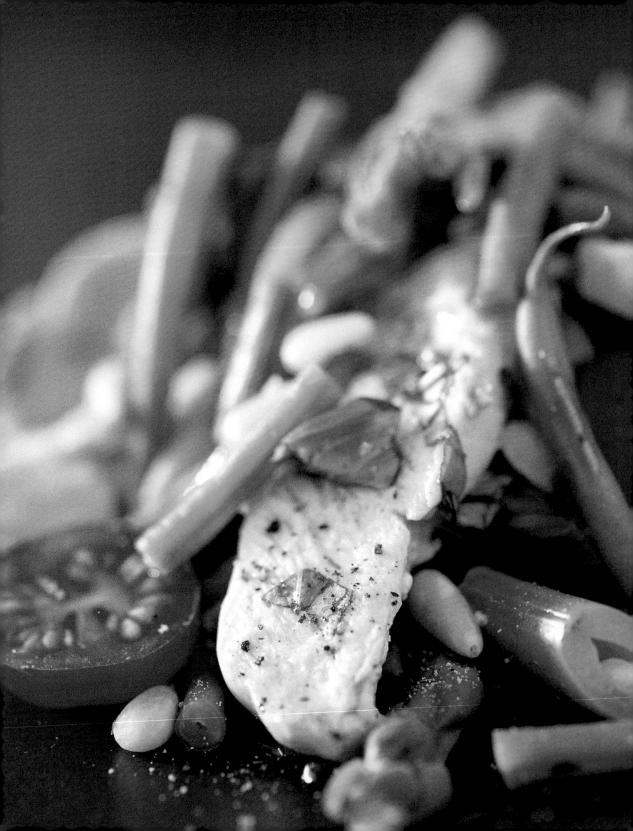

WARM CHICKEN SALAD

SERVES 4
2 skinless organic chicken breasts
3 ounces green beans, trimmed
3 ounces asparagus spears
6 cherry tomatoes, halved
2 tbsp pine nuts
¼ cup chopped fresh basil
1 handful baby salad leaves
Dressing:
2 tbsp extra virgin olive oil
1 tsp cider vinegar
1 tsp Dijon mustard

1. Place the chicken in a small pan of cold water, bring to a boil, then lower the heat and simmer for 8–10 minutes. Remove from the pan and allow to cool slightly. Alternatively, steam in a steamer.

2. Steam the green beans and asparagus spears until tender but still crisp; refresh in cold water.

3. Mix the beans and asparagus with all the other salad ingredients in a bowl except for the baby salad leaves.

4. Place the dressing ingredients in a screw-top jar with 1 tablespoon of water and shake well.

5. Slice the chicken while still warm and add to the salad. Pour over the dressing and toss to coat.

6. Serve in a large salad bowl, garnished with the baby salad leaves.

SALAD NIÇOISE

SERVES 4
4-ounce piece fresh tuna
1 bunch asparagus tips
1 head Boston lettuce
½ pound baby spinach leaves
2 tbsp black olives
¼ pound cherry tomatoes, halved
2 hard-boiled eggs, shelled and cut in quarters (optional)
Dressing:
1 tsp Dijon mustard
1 tbsp olive oil
2 tsp cider vinegar

1. Heat a griddle or nonstick pan over high heat until very hot. Add the tuna and sear for 2–3 minutes. With a spatula, turn the tuna over and cook for an additional 2–3 minutes.
2. Bring a small pan of water to a boil, add the asparagus, and cook for 2 minutes. Remove from the heat, drain, and refresh in plenty of cold water.
3. Arrange the lettuce leaves, spinach, olives, tomatoes, and asparagus tips on a platter. Break up the tuna and place on the leaves. Add the egg if using.
4. For the dressing, mix the mustard with 1 teaspoon of water, then whisk in the oil and vinegar. Drizzle over the salad and serve.

GRATED CARROT AND ZUCCHINI COLESLAW

SERVES 4

3 carrots, trimmed, peeled, and grated
2 zucchinis, trimmed and cut into
fine julienne (matchstick) strips or grated
2 spring onions, trimmed and diced

1 tsp cider vinegar
1 tbsp egg-free mayonnaise
2 tbsp pumpkin seeds

1. Mix the carrots, zucchini, courgettes and spring onions in a medium bowl.
2. Mix the cider vinegar with the mayonnaise and then mix in
with the coleslaw ingredients. Cover and chill until ready to serve.
3. Serve garnished with the pumpkin seeds.

CUCUMBER, DULSE, AND AVOCADO SALAD

Dulse is a seaweed that has a nutty flavor, a great
addition to salads.

SERVES 4

1 ounce dulse sea vegetable
2 avocados
1 cucumber, peeled and thinly sliced
1 carrot, trimmed, peeled and grated
¼ pound natural sauerkraut
1 handful chopped fresh chives

1 small bunch watercress, trimmed
and cut into bite-size pieces
2 tbsp freshly pressed apple juice
Zest of 1 lemon
Juice of half a lemon

1. Rinse the dulse in cold water and soak for 2–3 minutes.
Drain and squeeze out the excess water. Chop into bite-size pieces.
2. Peel and pit the avocados, and cut into small pieces.
3. Mix the dulse and avocado with all the other ingredients
in a large salad bowl and serve.

WARM RED LENTIL SALAD

Red lentils help strengthen the adrenal glands and kidneys. They are also a rich source of fiber, which makes them a great addition to any weight-loss program.

SERVES 4
¼ pound red lentils
2 shallots, peeled and chopped
1 garlic clove, peeled and crushed
1 tsp chopped fresh ginger
2 tsp wheat-free vegetable bouillon powder
¼ pound fresh mixed salad leaves, including arugula
and/or baby spinach leaves
2 tbsp chopped fresh cilantro or mint
4 lime wedges

1. Rinse and drain the lentils and place in a medium saucepan. Add the shallots, garlic, ginger, and bouillon powder and cover in cold water. Bring to a boil, then lower the heat and simmer for 10–15 minutes, or until tender. Stir occasionally.
2. Remove from the heat and drain away the excess water.
3. Divide the salad leaves among serving plates and pile the red lentils on top.
4. Garnish with the cilantro or mint and lime wedges (for squeezing) and serve.

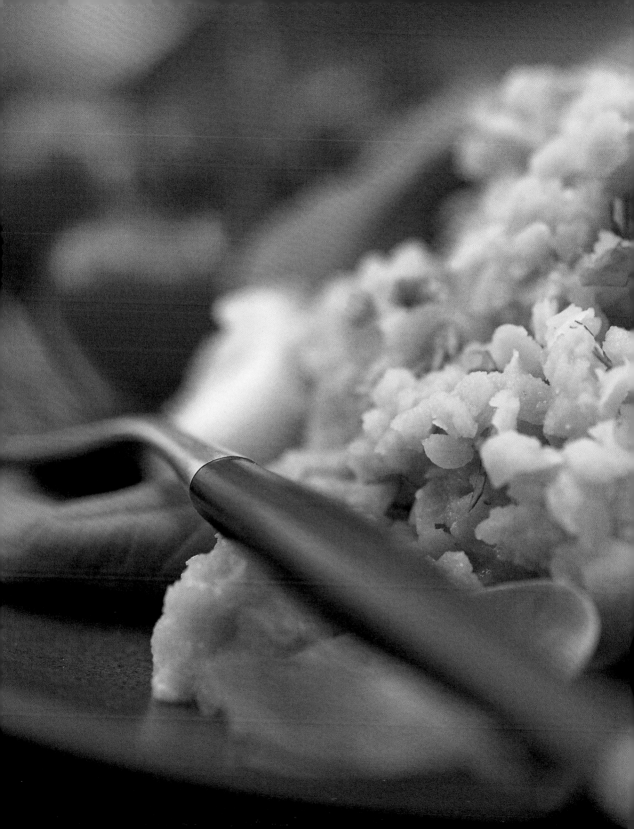

GREEN SALAD

SERVES 4

2 tbsp pine nuts
1 ripe avocado, pitted, peeled, and sliced
Half a cucumber, thinly sliced
1 celery stalk, trimmed and thinly sliced
¼ pound watercress
¼ pound arugula
1 baby Boston lettuce, leaves whole

Dressing:
1 tsp Dijon mustard
1 tbsp cider vinegar
2 tbsp olive oil

1. Place the pine nuts in a small pan over low heat and toast, stirring frequently, until golden in color. Set aside.
2. Mix the dressing ingredients together in a large salad bowl.
3. Add the avocado to the dressing and toss, then pile the other salad ingredients, except the pine nuts, on top.
4. Just before serving, toss the salad and sprinkle with the pine nuts.

SEAWEED SALAD

SERVES 4

2 ounces mixed seaweed
½ pound red or yellow cherry tomatoes, halved
2 spring onions, trimmed and thinly sliced
¼ pound arugula
1 endive
1 tbsp pumpkin seeds

Dressing:
1 tbsp cider vinegar
2 tsp pumpkin oil

1. Soak the seaweed for 10 minutes in cold water, then drain well.
2. Mix the seaweed with the tomatoes and spring onions. Place the arugula in a salad bowl and top with the seaweed mixture. Arrange the endive leaves around the edge of the salad.
3. Mix the dressing ingredients together and pour over the salad. Serve garnished with the pumpkin seeds.

WILD RICE SALAD WITH BEETS

SERVES 4

½ cup brown rice
½ cup wild rice
4 shallots, peeled and halved
2 tsp olive oil
4 cooked beets, diced

Juice of 1 lemon
2 tbsp chopped fresh mint
2 tbsp chopped fresh parsley
2 tbsp chopped fresh chives

1. Preheat the oven to 400°F.
2. Place the brown and wild rice in a medium pan of water. Bring to a boil, then lower the heat and simmer for 20 minutes.
3. Place the shallots in a small pan, cover with water, and bring to a boil. Cook for 2 minutes, remove from the heat and allow to cool, then drain.
4. Place the shallots on a baking sheet, drizzle with the oil, and roast for 5 minutes.
5. Drain the rice and allow to cool. Mix with the beets, lemon juice, and mint.
6. Stir in the shallots, parsley, and chives and serve.

BROCCOLI SALAD WITH APPLE VINAIGRETTE

SERVES 4

1 head broccoli, cut into florets
2 zucchinis, trimmed and cut into fine julienne (matchstick) strips
2 celery stalks, trimmed and cut on the diagonal
1 small bunch radishes, trimmed and quartered

Apple vinaigrette:
1 tbsp Dijon mustard
2 tbsp white miso paste or
1 tbsp wheat-free tamari
1 tsp toasted sesame oil
3 tbsp freshly pressed apple juice

1. Bring a medium saucepan of water to a boil. Add the broccoli and blanch for 2–3 minutes. Strain and run under cold water until completely cooled.
2. Place the broccoli in a salad bowl with the zucchini, celery, and radishes.
3. Place the vinaigrette ingredients in a screw-top jar and shake well to blend.
4. Pour the vinaigrette over the salad and serve.

GOAT CHEESE SALAD WITH ROASTED TOMATOES, PEPPERS, AND ARUGULA

Goat cheese is a good source of calcium, and also potassium, a mineral which helps to maintain normal blood pressure. Perhaps the greatest benefit is for people who cannot tolerate dairy products, most of whom are usually able to eat goat cheese without any problems. Enjoy this recipe as a special treat.

SERVES 4
4 red peppers, seeded and halved
12 cherry tomatoes
2 tsp olive oil
4 ounces goat cheese, crumbled
2 tbsp pine nuts
½ pound arugula
2 tbsp chopped fresh basil

1. Preheat the oven to 400°F.
2. Place the peppers (cut-side up) and tomatoes on a baking sheet, drizzle with the olive oil, and roast for 10 minutes. Sprinkle the goat cheese inside the peppers and cook for an additional 5 minutes.
3. Scatter over the pine nuts and return to the oven for 5 more minutes.
4. Arrange the arugula on 4 plates and top with the peppers and tomatoes. Serve garnished with the fresh basil.

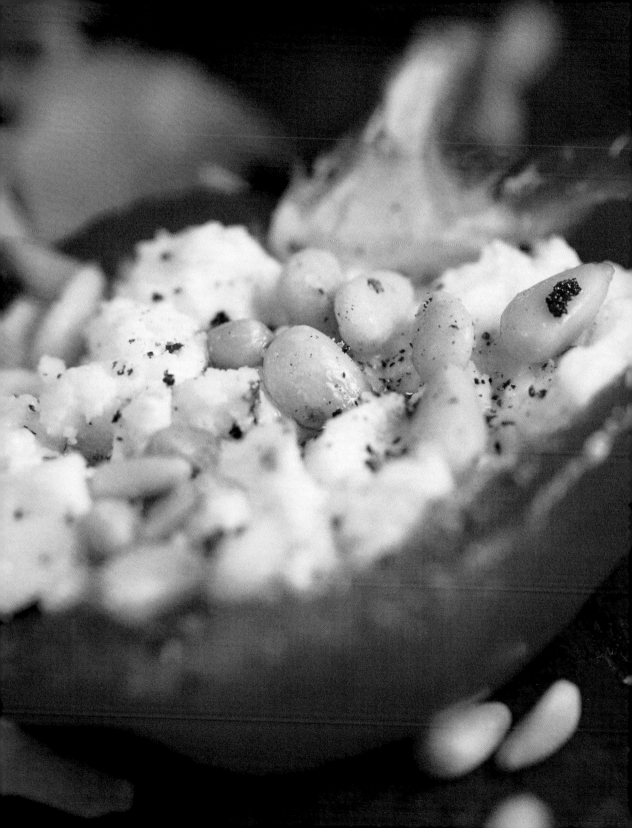

LUNCH-BOXES

After years of working with clients, I have found that there are two major issues that surround lunch: most people are at a loss as to what they should eat when it comes to lunch-time and many people simply eat lunch far too late in the day.

First, I want you to eat a lot of food at lunch time. Second, I want you to eat this ample lunch at roughly the same time each day for regulation of your internal body clock. Always eat your lunch sometime between noon and 1:30 p.m. at the latest, so that you don't disrupt your blood sugar—glucose balance. One of the biggest problems that I have found in practice is that clients often complain of massive energy slumps mid- or late afternoon. This is directly related to lunch—either they are not eating enough, they are eating sweets and junk food, or just waiting too long to eat and conjuring up excuses as to why there's no time.

Make the time to prepare for lunch and proper time to actually eat your lunch. Even if you have to get foods ready the night before, then so be it. It really will be worth it. Here we go with my easy lunch-box ideas.

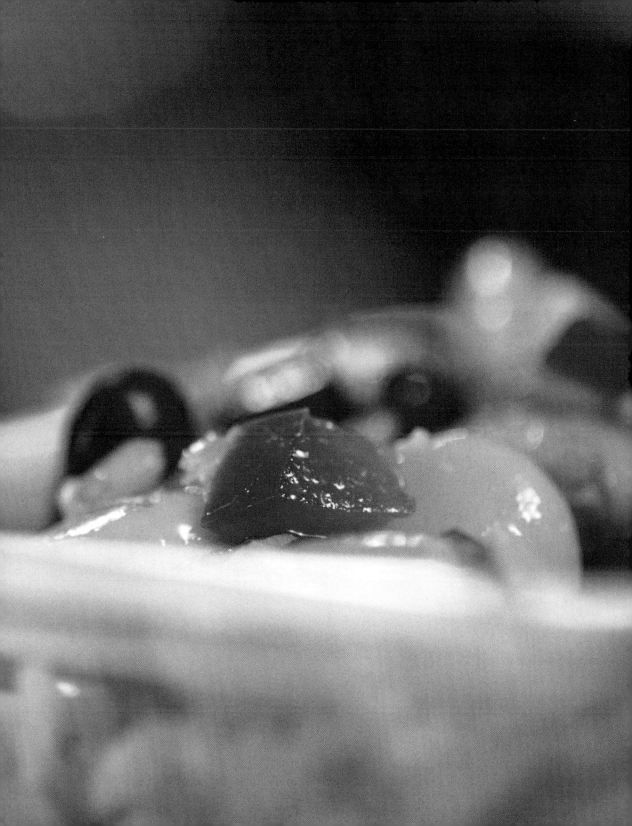

LUNCH-BOX OPTIONS

1

Bunch of red grapes (always eat your fruit first—it might
seem a bit strange initially, but your digestion will thank you)
Flask of soup (see pages 83–105)
Salad Niçoise (page 120) or make a simple salad of tuna,
hard-boiled egg (optional), baby spinach leaves, and green beans
Veggie crudités and Homemade Hummus (page 211)
Pumpkin seeds

2

Melon slices
Lima Bean Spread (page 205) with a variety of crunchy raw veggies
Corn on the cob (cook the night before and store in the fridge
in an airtight container)
Soaked almonds

3

Banana or small container of berries
Flask of soup
Wild Rice Salad (page 125)
Veggie crudités and Sesame Squash Spread (page 204)
Sunflower seeds

4

2 nectarines
Flask of soup
Toasted Nori Strips (page 213)
Sliced chicken breast with cherry tomatoes,
Arugula and Crunchy Walnut Coleslaw (page 111)
Hemp seeds and pumpkin seeds

5

Peach
Flask of soup
Couscous and Grated Carrot and Zucchini Coleslaw (page 121)
Rice cakes with Black Olive Tapenade (page 208)

CHAPTER 8 MAIN MEALS

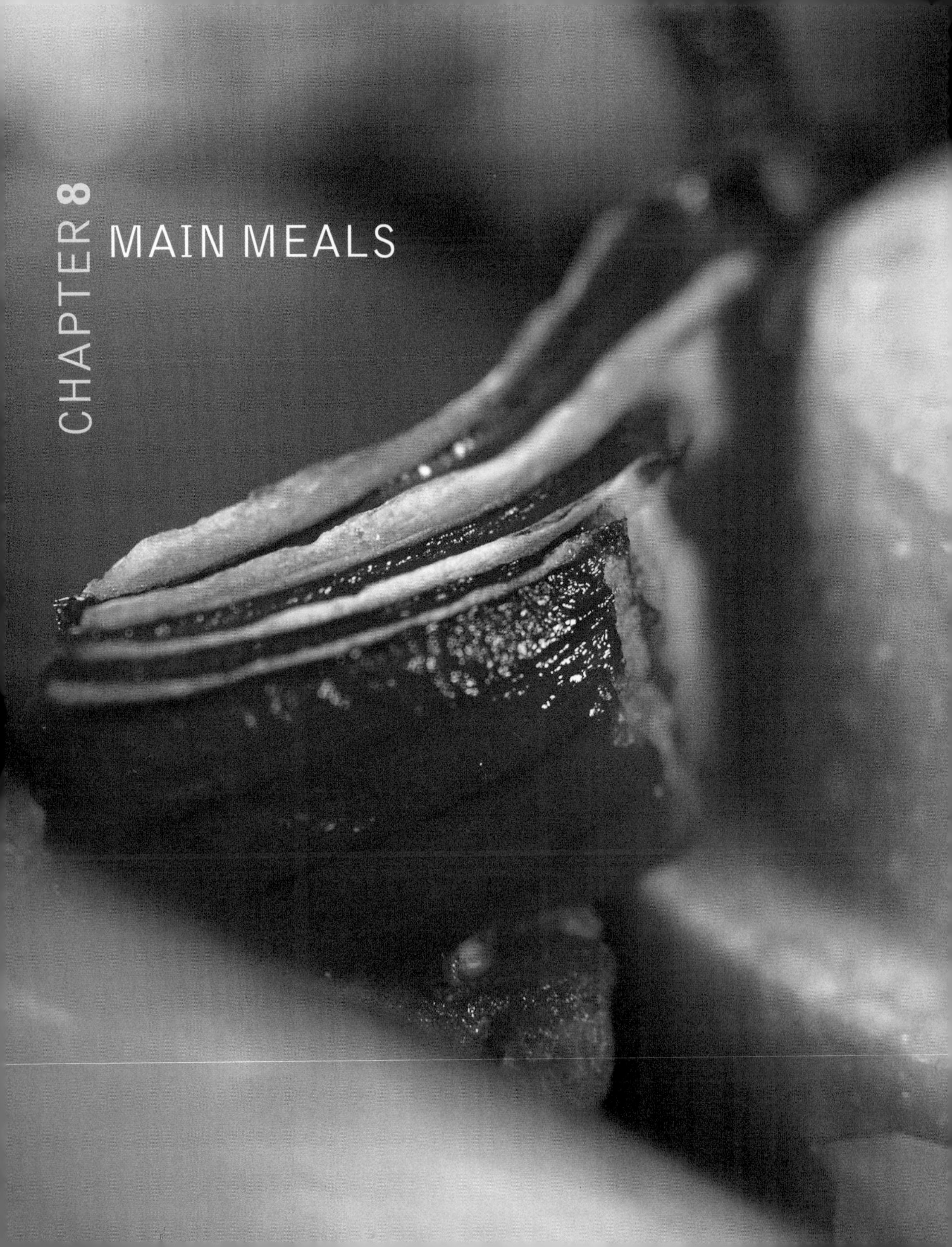

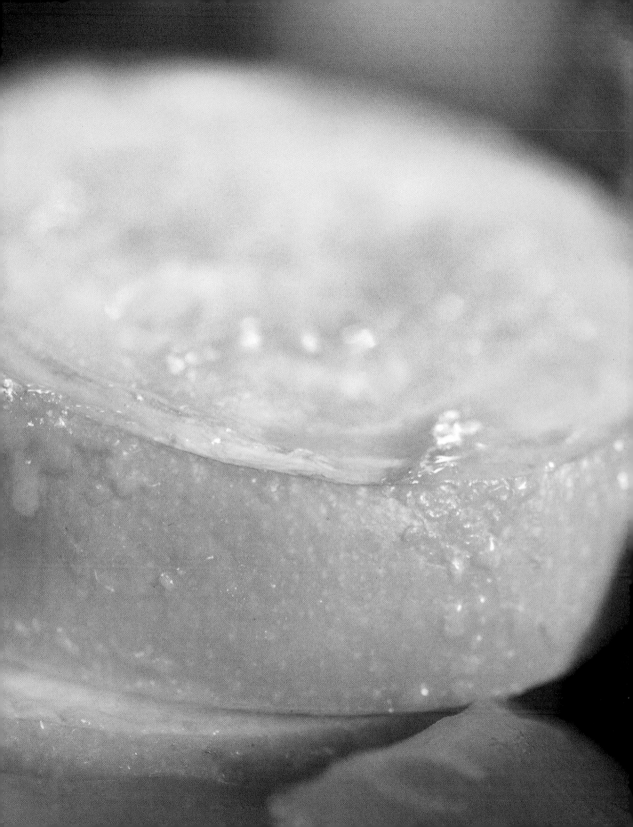

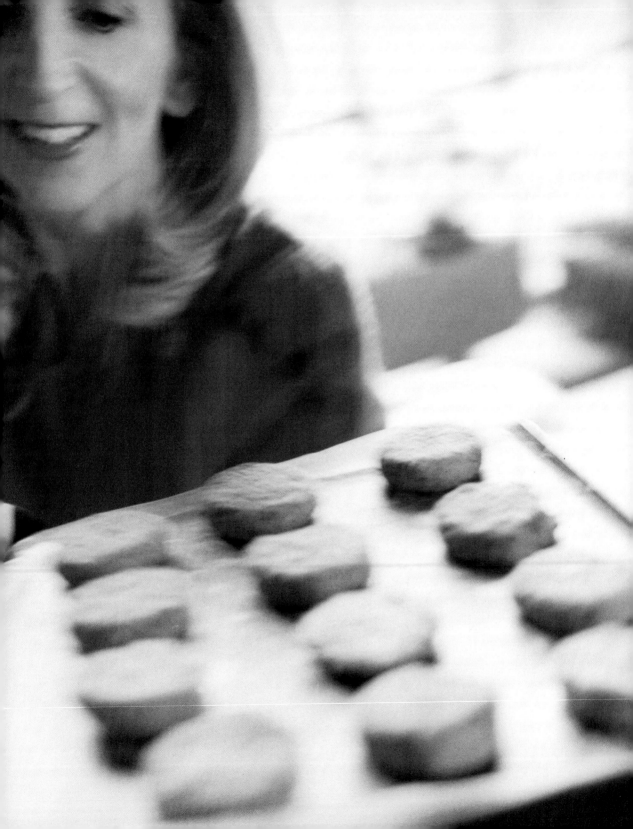

CHICKPEA BURGERS

These are a hit in any household. As well as making a meal in themselves, any mini-burgers left over can be used in a lunch-box or as a snack. Kids love them—and they're healthy too. Chickpeas have a naturally sweet flavor, are a good source of iron and good fats and nutritionally help out the tummy and heart. I have combined them with sunflower seeds—power-packed with EFAs, minerals, and B vitamins for an energy pick-me-up.

MAKES 20
16-ounce can chickpeas, drained and rinsed
16-ounce can kidney beans, drained and rinsed
1 carrot, trimmed, peeled, and finely grated
1 small onion, peeled and finely grated
½ cup sunflower seeds
2 tbsp tahini, drained of any excess oil before measuring
1 garlic clove, peeled and chopped
1 handful chopped fresh cilantro
1 tbsp wheat-free vegetable bouillon powder

1. Preheat the oven to 425°F. Line a large baking sheet with parchment paper.
2. Place all the ingredients in a food processor (or use a handheld blender) and blend for 5–10 seconds, until the mixture is fairly coarse. Push the mixture down with a spatula and blend for an additional 10 seconds.
3. Remove the blades from the processor, wet your hands under the cold water tap, and shape the mixture into 20 small balls.
4. Place the balls on the prepared baking sheet and flatten slightly with the back of the spoon.
5. Bake for 15–18 minutes, until lightly colored. Remove from the oven and allow to rest. Serve with Sweet Potato Wedges (see page 212) and a crunchy raw salad of snow peas, radishes, grated carrot, sliced celery, and fennel dressed with a squeeze of lemon juice.

CHICKEN BURGERS

Try to buy free-range, organic chicken.

MAKES 6
1 pound skinless organic chicken breasts, chilled
3 spring onions, trimmed and sliced
1 garlic clove, peeled and chopped
2 tbsp chopped fresh parsley
1 tsp organic wheat-free vegetable bouillon powder
2 heads baby Boston lettuce
½ pound cherry tomatoes, halved
1 carrot, trimmed, peeled, and grated
Half a cucumber, trimmed and sliced
Half a red pepper, trimmed, seeded, and sliced
Half a yellow pepper, trimmed, seeded, and sliced

1. Preheat the oven to 400°F. Line a baking sheet with aluminum foil.
2. Cut the chicken breasts into chunks, then place in a food processor and process for 1 minute. Add the spring onions, garlic, and parsley and blend for an additional 30 seconds.
3. Dissolve the bouillon powder in 1 tablespoon of hot water and add to the chicken mixture. Blend for 30 seconds to allow the mixture to form a soft ball.
4. Remove from the food processor and place in a clean bowl. Cover and chill for 30 minutes.
5. Wet your hands under the cold water tap and shape the mixture into 6 even-sized balls. Place on the prepared baking sheet and lightly press with the back of a spoon to form burger shapes.
6. Place in the preheated oven and bake for 5–7 minutes. Turn the burgers over and bake for an additional 5–10 minutes.
7. Remove from the oven and allow to rest for 5 minutes. Place each burger on two Boston lettuce leaves and top with tomatoes, grated carrot, and cucumber and pepper slices. Serve with my Tangy Barbecue Relish (see page 232).

STEAMED APPLE CHICKEN

This is a good transitional dish for people who are changing from really sweet, overly processed diets to a more wholesome diet. The extra sweetness provided by the apple juice facilitates the changeover. It's best served with bean sprouts for a boost of energy-giving food enzymes that also help improve digestion.

SERVES 4

4 skinless organic chicken breasts
2 tsp avocado or olive oil
1½-inch piece fresh ginger, peeled and finely chopped
2 garlic cloves, peeled and chopped
2 small onions, peeled and diced
2 carrots, trimmed, peeled, and diced
1 small red pepper, seeded and diced
1 head broccoli, cut into small florets
20 baby corn, trimmed
1 cup freshly pressed apple juice
¼ pound raw bean sprouts

1. Preheat the oven to 400°F.
2. Take a large piece of aluminum foil and place the chicken breasts in the center. Drizzle over the oil and add the ginger, garlic, and vegetables. Draw up the sides of the foil and pour in the apple juice.
3. Scrunch up the foil to seal everything in and place in the oven for 10–15 minutes.
4. Remove from the oven and allow to rest for 5 minutes.
5. Transfer the foil parcels to four serving plates, open the parcels slightly, and serve immediately with the raw bean sprouts and a large salad.

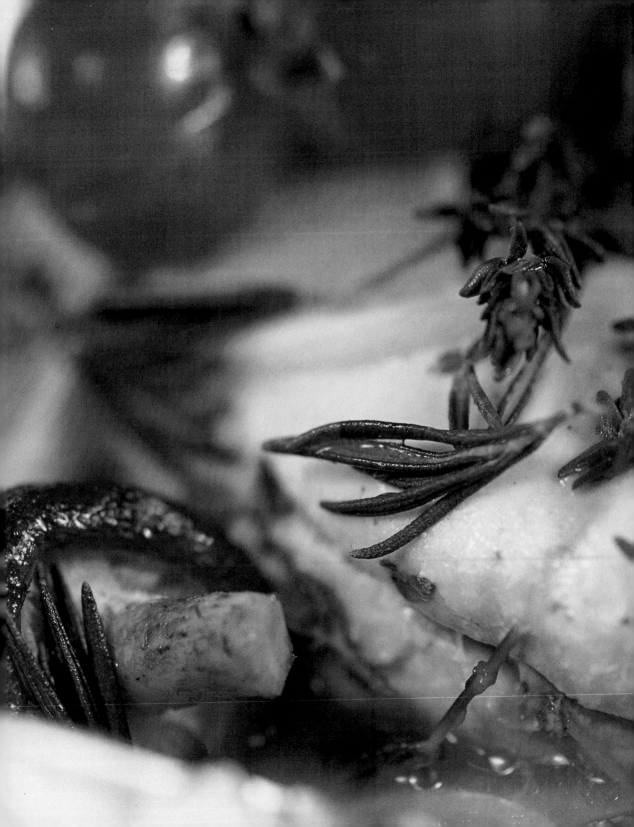

BAKED BUTTERFLIED CHICKEN WITH SHIITAKE MUSHROOMS

In this dish, I have used one of the most healing foods around: Shiitake mushrooms are a superb immune system tonic. Even people who suffer from yeasty conditions and normally have to avoid mushrooms can eat shiitakes, as they contain substances that can lower nasty yeasties and bacteria.

SERVES 4
1 tbsp olive oil
4 skinless organic chicken breasts
¼ pound shiitake mushrooms, trimmed
1 garlic clove, peeled and chopped
4 shallots, peeled and finely chopped
2 tbsp chopped fresh parsley
1 tbsp wheat-free vegetable bouillon powder dissolved in ½ cup hot water
12 cherry tomatoes
4 small sprigs fresh thyme
4 small sprigs fresh rosemary
1 lemon, cut into 4 wedges

1. Preheat the oven to 400°F.
2. Take a large piece of aluminum foil and oil the center of the foil with a pastry brush.
3. With a sharp knife, carefully slice through the center of the chicken breasts horizontally to form a pocket. Do not cut all the way through.
4. Fill the pockets with the mushrooms, garlic, shallots, and parsley. Place on the oiled foil, draw up the sides, and add the bouillon water, 3 cherry tomatoes, and 1 sprig each of thyme and rosemary. Squeeze with lemon.
5. Scrunch up the foil to seal everything in and place on a baking sheet in the oven for 10–15 minutes.
6. Remove from the oven and allow to rest in the foil for 5 minutes.
7. Transfer the foil parcels to four serving plates, open the parcels slightly, and serve immediately with a large salad.

TEMPEH WITH KALE, RADISHES, AND SAUERKRAUT

Kale is an exceptional source of chlorophyll, iron, calcium, and other minerals, a superveg. I often use radishes in soups, too, to help prevent colds and clear the sinuses. And my favorite, sauerkraut, is very good for the liver.

SERVES 4
3 ounces tempeh
1 strip kombu sea vegetable
2 tsp tamari sauce
1-inch piece fresh ginger, peeled and thinly sliced
½ pound curly kale
1 tsp olive oil
1 small bunch radishes, trimmed and cut in half
3–4 tbsp natural sauerkraut
1 tbsp pumpkin seeds

1. Cut the tempeh into 4 pieces and place in a medium pan with the kombu, tamari sauce, and ginger. Pour in enough water to half-cover the tempeh. Bring to a boil, then lower the heat and simmer for 10 minutes. Remove from the heat and allow to cool.
2. Bring a medium pan of water to a boil, add the kale, and boil for 3–4 minutes. Drain and rinse in cold water.
3. Strain and slice the tempeh, discarding the kombu and ginger.
4. Heat the oil in a small skillet with 1 tablespoon of water, add the tempeh, and pan-fry for a few seconds.
5. Arrange the kale, radishes, and sauerkraut on a serving platter, top with the tempeh, and serve garnished with the pumpkin seeds.

THE McKEITH SHEPHERDESS PIE

This is a big favorite of many of the participants on my TV program, *You Are What You Eat*. Root veggies strengthen and improve digestion by lowering the amount of acidity in the body and stimulating the growth of healthy gut flora. Always be sure to serve with plenty of raw salad leaves.

SERVES 4

4 sweet potatoes, peeled and roughly chopped
2 tsp olive oil
1 garlic clove, peeled and crushed
2 celery stalks, trimmed and thinly sliced
1 onion, peeled and thinly sliced
¾ pound butternut squash, peeled, seeded, and chopped into bite-size pieces
2 cups Roasted Vegetable Stock (see page 230)

16-ounce can kidney beans, drained and rinsed
16-ounce can black-eyed peas, drained and rinsed
2 red peppers, seeded and sliced
2 zucchinis, trimmed and sliced
4 tomatoes, sliced in half
2 tsp arrowroot powder
2 tbsp chopped fresh parsley

1. Preheat the oven to 400°F.
2. Steam or boil the sweet potatoes for 10–15 minutes, until completely tender.
3. Place 2 tablespoons of water in a medium saucepan with the oil, garlic, celery, and onion and cook for 3 minutes. Add the squash and cook for an addtional 2 minutes, stirring frequently. Add the stock and bring to a boil. Cover, lower the heat, and simmer for 10 minutes.
4. Add the beans, peas, peppers, zucchini, and tomatoes and simmer for an addtional 5 minutes.
5. Mix the arrowroot with a little water and add along with the parsley.
6. Drain the sweet potatoes and mash.
7. Transfer the filling to a pie dish and top with the mashed sweet potatoes.
8. Bake for 12–15 minutes, until the sweet potato begins to brown. Serve immediately with a green salad.

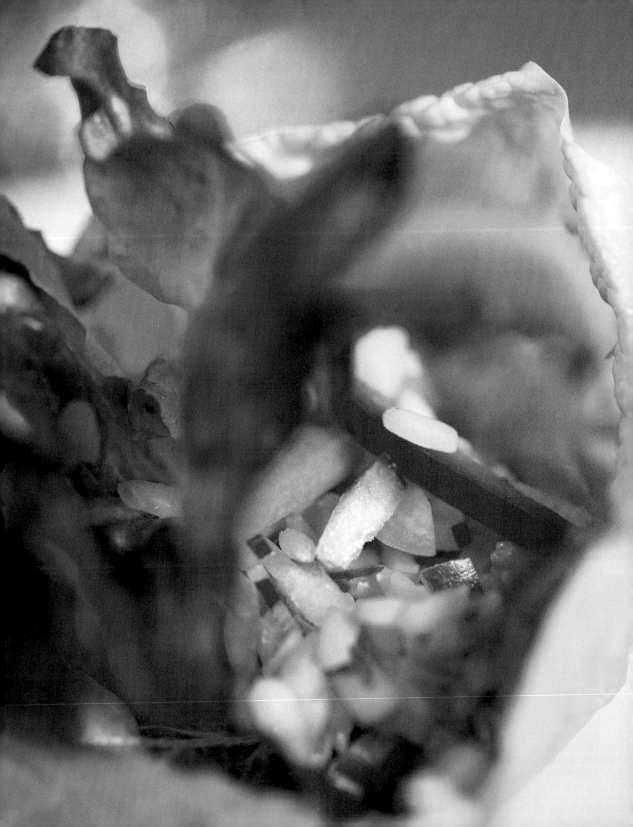

LETTUCE AND CASHEW WRAPS
WITH TAHINI DRESSING

Lettuce is great on a weight-loss program because it's a diuretic. It's also a calming food and can even help dry up dampness in the body caused by yeast and bacteria brought on by poor digestion. Have a look at your tongue in the mirror. If there's a white or yellow coating, a line down the middle, or cuts or serrations at the very back, then it's lettuce to the rescue.

These wraps are also perfect for packed lunches (see page 130). Try some of your own fillings—chopped cooked chicken or flaked tuna make good alternatives to the cashews.

MAKES 6

Dressing:
3 tbsp tahini
1 tbsp cider vinegar

Optional:
Hummus

6 large lettuce leaves (romaine, iceberg, or oak leaf)
1 carrot, trimmed, peeled, and cut into fine julienne (matchstick) strips
1 red pepper, seeded and thinly sliced
2 spring onions, trimmed and thinly sliced
2 tbsp chopped red onion
½ cup cashews, roughly chopped
3 ounces bean sprouts
2 tbsp tamari sauce

1. Prepare the dressing by mixing the tahini and cider vinegar together with 3 tablespoons of cold water in a small mixing bowl.
2. Arrange the salad leaves on a large platter.
3. In a bowl, mix together all the other ingredients and divide among the lettuce leaves. Spoon a little of the dressing over the filling. Roll the leaves around the filling and secure with a toothpick.
4. Serve the wraps with the remaining dressing on the side.

NAVY BEAN LOAF

Navy beans are an excellent source of protein and support kidney-adrenal function, metabolism, and regulation of blood sugar levels.

SERVES 4
2 tsp olive oil
1 leek, washed, trimmed, and sliced
1-inch piece fresh ginger, peeled and grated
½ tsp ground cumin
½ tsp ground coriander
1 onion, peeled and quartered
3 carrots, trimmed, peeled, and grated
1 garlic clove, peeled and chopped
3 tbsp chopped fresh parsley
½ cup sunflower seeds
½ cup oat bran
1 tbsp wheat-free vegetable bouillon powder
16-ounce can navy beans, drained and rinsed
16-ounce can cannellini beans, drained and rinsed

1. Preheat the oven to 375°F. Lightly oil a loaf pan and line the base with parchment paper.
2. Put the remaining oil and the leek in a small saucepan and cook over low heat for 5 minutes. Add the ginger, cumin, and coriander and cook for an additional minute. Remove from the heat and allow to cool.
3. Place the onion, carrots, garlic, parsley, sunflower seeds, oat bran, bouillon powder, and one of the cans of beans (either will do) in a food processor and blend for 20 seconds, or until semi-smooth. Transfer to a large bowl and stir in the second, can of beans and the leek mixture.
4. Spoon into the prepared pan and bake for 40–45 minutes, until golden brown in color.
5. Turn out of the pan onto a serving plate. Serve either hot or cold with a lightly dressed salad.

MEDITERRANEAN BLACK-EYED PEA CASSEROLE

A fantastic adrenal-strengthener and fiber-rich meal.

SERVES 4
1 tbsp olive oil
1 garlic clove, peeled and finely chopped
2 onions, peeled and thinly sliced
16-ounce can black-eyed peas, drained and rinsed
3 tomatoes, quartered
¼ pound shiitake mushrooms, trimmed and quartered
2 carrots, trimmed, peeled, and diced
1 tbsp chopped fresh basil
1 tsp dried oregano
1 tsp dried marjoram
2 tsp tamari sauce
2 zucchinis, trimmed and cut into fine julienne (matchstick) strips
1 tsp capers (optional)
1 tbsp each chopped fresh basil, oregano, and parsley

1. Heat the oil in a medium casserole dish on the stovetop. Add the garlic and onions and cook for a couple of minutes. Add the peas, tomatoes, mushrooms, carrots, dried herbs, and tamari. Bring to a boil, then lower the heat and simmer for 10–15 minutes. When cooked, the vegetables should still have a little bite. Add a little water or stock if needed during the cooking process.

2. Remove from the heat and add the zucchini. Serve from the casserole dish and garnish with the capers, if using, and the fresh herbs. Accompany with Gourmet Brown Rice (see page 195) and a side salad.

BAKED SALMON WITH SPINACH AND LEEKS

More than two-thirds of the people who come to see me for the first time test deficient in omega-3 fats. This dish provides plenty through the avocado and salmon.

SERVES 4
2 leeks, washed, trimmed, and sliced
1 pound fresh baby spinach leaves
Four 4-ounce organic salmon fillets
1 tbsp olive oil
2 garlic cloves, peeled and finely chopped
1 tbsp grated fresh ginger
Juice of half a lemon
1 handful fresh cilantro leaves, to garnish

1. Preheat the oven to 400°F.
2. Gently boil or steam the leeks for 5 minutes to soften.
3. Place the spinach leaves in a medium baking pan and top with the leeks. Place the salmon on top.
4. Mix together the oil, garlic, and ginger and liberally brush over the salmon using a pastry brush. Pour over the lemon juice.
5. Place in the oven and bake for 10 minutes. Remove and allow to rest for 5 minutes. Garnish with the fresh cilantro leaves and serve with Avocado Dressing (see page 161) drizzled over the top.

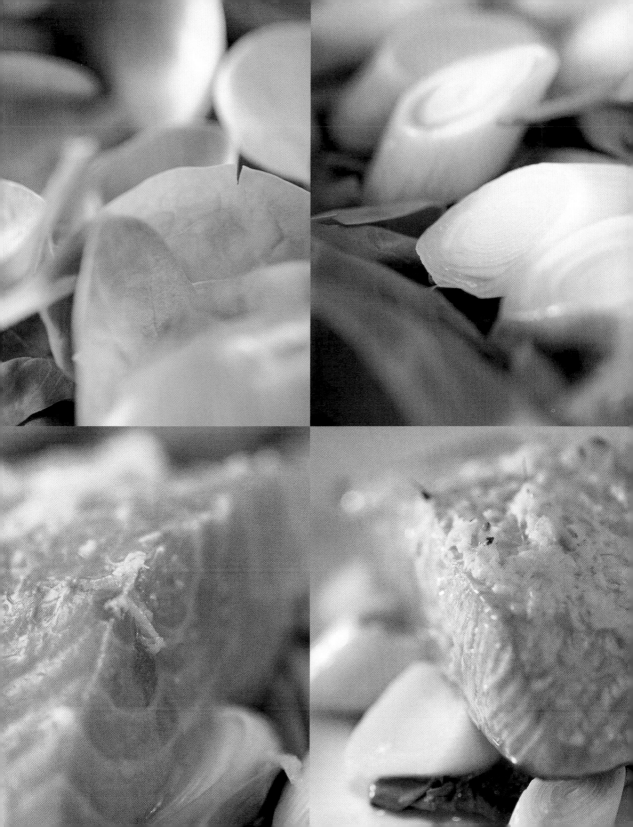

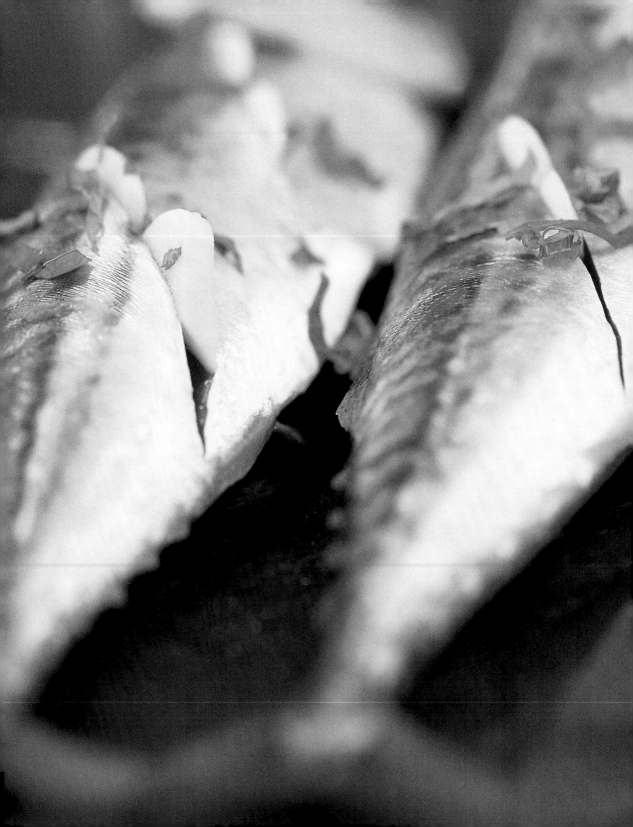

MACKEREL WITH PINE NUTS AND PARSLEY

Many of us don't get nearly enough good fats in our diet, and they are plentiful in this recipe. Pine nuts are also helpful to the lungs, colon, and intestines, while parsley is an herbal "multivitamin" and excellent for good digestion. What more could you possibly ask for in a dish?

SERVES 4

4 whole mackerel, scaled and gutted
1 garlic clove, peeled and sliced
¼ cup chopped fresh parsley
8 lemon slices
Filling:
4 spring onions, trimmed and chopped
3 tbsp roughly chopped pine nuts
3 tbsp chopped fresh parsley
Zest of 1 lemon
1 garlic clove, peeled and chopped

Garnish:
1 handful mixed salad leaves
6 cherry tomatoes, halved
Quarter of a cucumber sliced
Half a yellow pepper, seeded and thinly sliced
4 lemon wedges

1. Preheat the broiler to high. Cover the broiler pan with aluminum foil.
2. With a sharp knife, make two incisions in the side of each mackerel. Fill the incisions with garlic and parsley and place on the pan.
3. Combine the filling ingredients together in a small bowl and use to stuff the cavity of the fish.
4. Arrange the lemon slices over the fish. Place under the hot broiler and cook for 3–4 minutes. Turn the mackerel over and repeat on the second side.
5. Remove from under the broiler and allow the fish to rest for 5 minutes. Divide the salad garnish ingredients and lemon wedges (for squeezing) among 4 plates, add the mackerel, and serve.

BAKED FISH WITH CARROT AND LEEK PURÉE

Leeks are in the same family as onions and garlic and so have the same health benefits, including anti-cancer properties, helping lower "bad" cholesterol (LDL), while raising "good" cholesterol (HDL) and stabilizing blood sugar levels.

SERVES 4
4 carrots, trimmed, peeled, and sliced
1 leek, washed, trimmed, and sliced
1 tbsp wheat-free vegetable bouillon powder
Four 4-ounce white fish fillets, such as haddock or whiting
4 tsp olive oil, plus extra to glaze
¼ pound fresh garden peas
2 tbsp chopped fresh mint
¼ pound watercress
¼ pound arugula

1. Preheat the oven to 400°F.
2. Place the carrots and leek in a medium to large saucepan. Add the bouillon powder and enough boiling water to cover. Bring back to a boil, then lower the heat and simmer for approximately 10–15 minutes, or until tender when pierced with a knife. Allow to cool slightly, then blend in a food processor or with a handheld blender until smooth.
3. Line a baking sheet with aluminum foil and place the fish on it, evenly spaced. Using a pastry brush, glaze the fish with olive oil.
4. Transfer to the oven and bake for 8–10 minutes.
5. Bring a small pan of water to a boil and add the peas. Cook for 2–3 minutes, then drain, reserving about 1 tablespoon of the juice. Add the 4 tsp oil and the mint and crush the peas with the back of a fork.
6. Take 4 warmed serving plates and divide the purée among them. Place the fish on the purée and then spoon the pea mixture on top. Garnish with the watercress and arugula and serve immediately.

SALMON WITH ORANGE AND SOY SAUCE

SERVES 4
¼ cup tamari sauce
Zest and juice of 1 orange
1-inch piece fresh ginger, peeled and finely chopped
1 garlic clove, peeled and crushed
4 spring onions, trimmed and sliced
Four 6-ounce organic salmon fillets
1 orange, thinly sliced
½ pound mixed baby spinach, watercress, and arugula leaves

1. Preheat the oven to 400°F.
2. Mix together the tamari, zest and juice of the orange, ginger, garlic, and spring onions in a shallow glass ovenproof pie dish. Add the salmon, cover in plastic wrap, and marinate in the fridge for 30 minutes, turning occasionally.
3. Uncover the dish and arrange the orange slices on the top.
4. Bake for 10–15 minutes, until the fish is firm to touch. Remove from the oven and allow to stand for 5 minutes.
5. Arrange the salad leaves on the plates and top with the salmon. Pour over the cooking juices. Serve with lightly steamed vegetables.

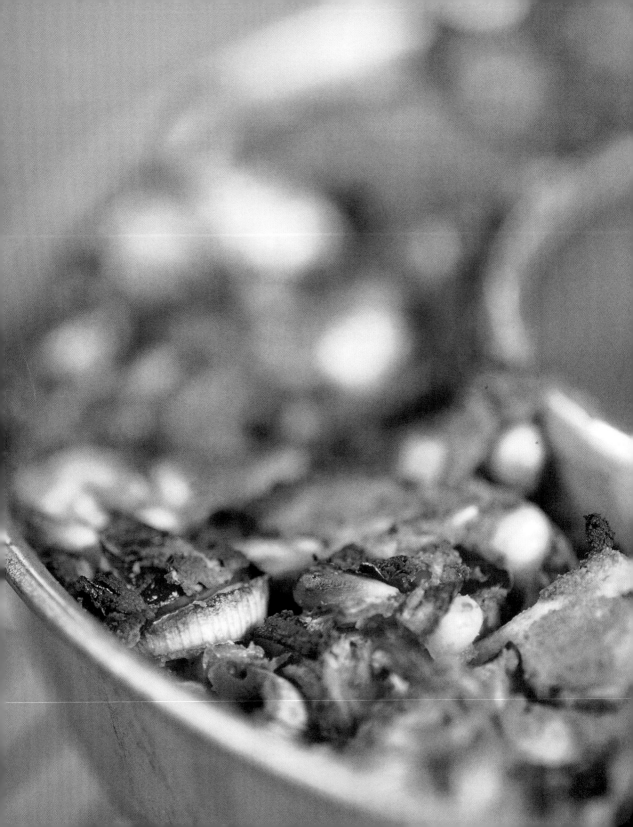

CHESTNUT ROAST

This recipe is perfect for the weekend or a special occasion.

SERVES 4

1 tbsp olive oil, plus extra to grease the pan
1 large red onion, peeled and finely chopped
3 garlic cloves, peeled and crushed
1 large leek, washed, trimmed, and sliced
2 carrots, trimmed, peeled, and sliced
1 large parsnip, trimmed, peeled, and chopped
8 ounces vacuum-packed chestnuts

¾ cup pine nuts
3 tbsp chopped fresh parsley
2 tbsp chopped fresh thyme
2 tsp finely chopped fresh rosemary
2 tsp wheat-free vegetable bouillon powder
4 ounces soft mild goat cheese (optional)
Fresh rosemary sprigs and bay leaves

1. Preheat the oven to 350°F.

2. Take a 9-inch round cake pan and use it to cut out a circle of parchment paper. Cut a hole in the center of the paper 1 inch larger than the hole in the pan. Make ½ inch cuts, 1½ inches apart, around the inside and outside of the paper circle. Brush the pan with a little olive oil, line with the paper, and brush with a little more oil.

3. Heat 1 tablespoon olive oil in a large skillet. Gently cook the onion and garlic for 3–5 minutes, stirring occasionally, until softened but not colored. Add the leek, carrots, and parsnip with 1½ cups water. Bring to a boil, then lower the heat and simmer for 6–8 minutes. The water will have evaporated and the vegetables should be tender when pierced with a knife. Allow to cool in the pan for 10 minutes.

4. Place the chestnuts in the food processor and blend for 10–15 seconds, until roughly chopped. Transfer to a large bowl and add the vegetables, pine nuts, parsley, thyme, rosemary, and bouillon powder. Mix well and spoon half the mixture into the prepared pan, pressing down well. Dot with half the cheese, if using, and then top with the remaining vegetable mixture. Dot with the rest of the cheese.

5. Bake for 40–45 minutes, until lightly browned. Remove from the oven and allow to cool in the pan for 5 minutes. Carefully loosen with a palette knife and turn out on to a warmed serving plate. Garnish with the fresh rosemary sprigs and bay leaves.

NAVY BEAN AND ROOT VEGETABLE STEW

A good source of fiber and those important B vitamins that are necessary for weight management and strong nervous systems.

SERVES 4
1 tbsp olive oil
2 onions, peeled and diced
2 bay leaves
Half a rutabaga, trimmed, peeled, and diced
3 carrots, trimmed, peeled, and cut into large chunks
Half a red pepper, seeded and thinly sliced
16-ounce can navy beans, drained and rinsed
½ tsp cumin seeds
1 tbsp white miso paste
2 tbsp chopped fresh parsley
2 ounces bean sprouts
4 spring onions, trimmed and thinly sliced

1. Heat a large casserole dish and add the oil, onions, bay leaves, and a little water. Cook for 10 minutes, until soft but not colored. Add the rutabaga, carrots, and pepper and enough water to cover. Bring to a boil, then reduce the heat and simmer gently for 10 minutes.

2. Stir in the beans, cumin, and white miso and simmer for an additional 10 minutes.

3. Serve immediately, garnished with the parsley, bean sprouts, and spring onions.

SMOKED TOFU AND BEAN BURGERS

Kidney beans are a good source of iron, magnesium, and folate. This recipe makes six chunky burgers that are ideal for a light lunch for six, or eight smaller burgers that would make a more generous meal for four people. Serve your burgers with one of my delicious raw side salads or some raw veggies. Never forget to do that. With every dish that is cooked, you need to complement it with some raw vegetables, leaves, or herbs to aid digestion and foods enzymes into the body.

MAKES 6–8

1 onion, peeled and quartered
1 garlic clove, peeled and chopped
1 carrot, trimmed, peeled, and grated
16-ounce can kidney beans, drained and rinsed

8 ounces smoked tofu, cut in 1-inch cubes
½ cup sunflower seeds
1 small bunch fresh parsley
2 tsp wheat-free vegetable bouillon powder

1. Preheat the oven to 400°F. Line a baking sheet with parchment paper.
2. Place all the ingredients in a food processor and blend for 6–8 minutes, until the mixture is roughly chopped but not smooth.
3. Remove the blade from the processor, take handfuls of the mixture, and shape into medium-size balls. Place on the baking sheet and press down gently with the back of a spoon to form burger shapes. You should get between 6 and 8 burgers, depending on the size of the burger.
4. Transfer to the oven and bake for 25 minutes, or until golden brown in color. Serve with a crispy green salad and Tangy Barbecue Relish (see page 232).

RISOTTO RICE

Rice is a fantastic source of those all-important B vitamins that are essential for the breakdown of proteins, fats, and carbs in the body as well as being a good stress-buster.

SERVES 4
1 cup risotto rice
2 tbsp wild rice
4 tsp olive oil
3 onions, peeled and diced
1 fennel bulb, trimmed, thinly sliced, and cored
½ cup rice milk
¼ pound baby corn
¼ pound cherry tomatoes, halved
6 tbsp chopped fresh basil

1. Mix the rices together, rinse, and place in a medium pan with 2 cups water. Bring to a boil, then lower the heat and simmer for 25–30 minutes, until all the liquid is absorbed. The rice should be cooked but slightly firm.
2. Heat the olive oil in a medium pan with 2 tablespoons of water and add the onions, fennel, and rice milk. Cook for 10 minutes, until the onion is soft but not colored.
3. Stir this mixture through the rice along with the remaining ingredients and serve immediately on a bed of curly endive, baby spinach, and arugula leaves.

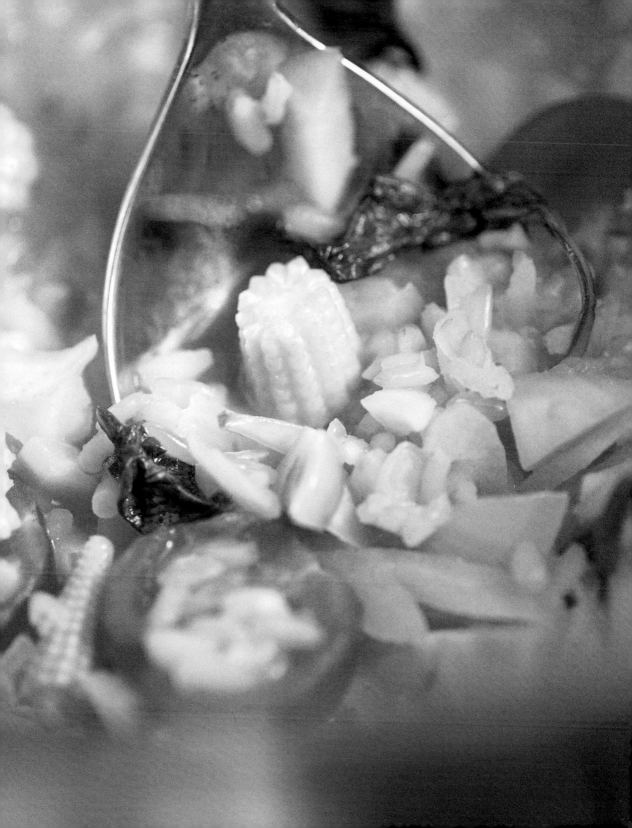

ADZUKI BEAN STEW

If you want to lose weight, this is the dish for you. As well as being great for weight loss, adzuki beans also contain high levels of B vitamins to nourish the adrenal glands and iron, zinc, and manganese, all of which are excellent for general health. They strengthen the body's energy battery, the spleen, and soak up damp in the body like a sponge.

SERVES 4
½ pound adzuki beans, soaked for 12 hours or overnight in cold water
1 wheat-free vegetable stock cube
1 onion, peeled and finely chopped
2 carrots, trimmed, peeled, and thickly sliced
1 leek, washed, trimmed, and thinly sliced
Half a butternut squash, peeled, halved, seeded, and cut into chunks
1 tsp ground cumin
1 tsp turmeric powder
½ pound curly kale, chopped
¼ cup chopped fresh chervil

1. Drain the beans and rinse well. Place in a large saucepan of water and bring to a boil. Boil hard for 15 minutes to remove the toxins. Drain and rinse well.

2. Return the beans to the pan with 1 quart of fresh cold water. Add the stock cube and bring to a boil. Lower the heat and simmer for 10 minutes. Add the vegetables, cumin, and turmeric and simmer for an additional 10–15 minutes.

3. Add the kale and cook for a few minutes, until just tender. Sprinkle with chervil and serve with Millet Mash (see page 159) and Onion Gravy (see page 229).

MILLET MASH

If you are a potato addict and are missing your buttery and milky mashed white potatoes, then this dish is going to make your day. Too many white potatoes in your diet can have an acidifying effect on your body, due to the fast energy glucose release that they cause. Millet, by contrast, supports the digestive organs, helps to improve nutrient uptake, and aids in the removal of unwanted excess acid from years of poor eating. To top it all, it also helps to inhibit the growth of fungus and nasty bacteria.

SERVES 4
½ cup millet
1 pinch of sea salt
1 onion, peeled and finely chopped
1 head cauliflower, cut into small florets

1. Wash the millet and drain well. Place in a medium pan of water, add the salt, and bring to a boil. Lower the heat and simmer for 20 minutes.
2. Place the onion in a medium pan with the cauliflower and enough water to cover. Bring to a boil, then lower the heat and simmer for 4–5 minutes. Remove from the heat, drain, and return to the pan. Mash with a potato masher.
3. Drain the millet and mix through the mashed cauliflower and onion mixture. Serve warm.

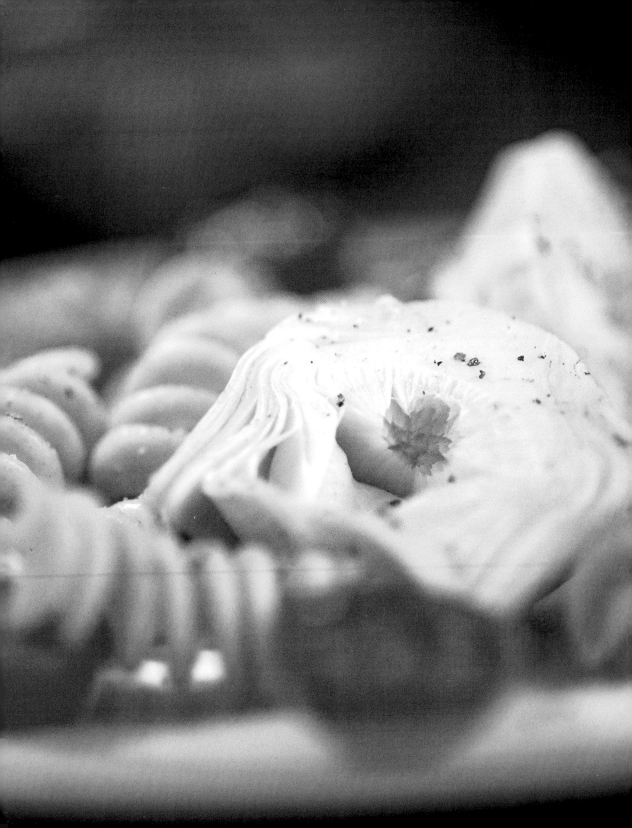

CHERRY TOMATO AND ARTICHOKE PASTA WITH AVOCADO DRESSING

I want to take the opportunity here today to tell you to stop eating processed white pasta. Instead, check out other types of pastas: spelt, yellow corn, or rice pasta and quinoa pasta too. You can find all kinds of varieties in your local health food store. In this dish, I use an ingredient called umeboshi paste, which is a fantastic way to flavor a dish. It's also a superb digestive tonic.

SERVES 4
$\frac{1}{2}$ pound wheat-free pasta
4 ounces marinated artichokes
$\frac{1}{2}$ pound cherry tomatoes, halved
$\frac{1}{2}$ cup chopped fresh basil, plus extra to garnish
Avocado dressing:
2 avocados, halved and pitted
Juice of 1 lemon
1 garlic clove, peeled and chopped
1 tbsp white miso paste
1 tsp umeboshi paste
1 tbsp olive oil

1. Bring a medium pan of water to a boil, add the pasta, and cook for 3–4 minutes, until al dente (just cooked); it will not take long, so don't overcook it. Drain and rinse well under cold water.
2. To make the dressing, scoop the flesh from the avocados into a small food processor bowl. Add all the other dressing ingredients and blend until smooth. If necessary, add a little cold water in order to form a smooth paste.
3. Mix together the pasta, artichokes, tomatoes, and the chopped basil.
4. Serve with the avocado dressing drizzled over the top, garnished with the extra basil.

EGGPLANT AND CHICKPEA TAGINE

A tagine is a Moroccan casserole dish designed to maximize flavor and retain nutrients. If you don't have a tagine, then a normal casserole dish will do fine.

SERVES 4
1 tbsp olive oil
2 onions, peeled and chopped
2 celery stalks, trimmed and sliced
1 small leek, washed, trimmed, and sliced
2 garlic cloves, peeled and finely chopped
1 tsp ground cumin
1 tsp ground coriander
1 tsp cinnamon
16-ounce can chopped organic tomatoes
1 large eggplant, cut into 1-inch pieces
2 small red peppers, seeded and diced
2 small yellow peppers, seeded and diced
1 tbsp wheat-free vegetable bouillon powder
16-ounce can chickpeas, drained and rinsed
1 handful fresh basil leaves
1 handful fresh cilantro leaves

1. Place the oil in a tagine or covered casserole dish and warm gently over low heat. Add the onions, celery, leek, and garlic and cook for 2 minutes. Add all the spices, the tomatoes, and vegetables and cook for an additional 3 minutes.
2. Mix the bouillon with 2 tablespoons of boiling water and add to the tagine.
3. Lower the heat and simmer for 40–50 minutes.
4. Add the chickpeas and cook for an additional 5 minutes.
5. Add the fresh herbs and serve from the tagine or casserole dish with brown rice.

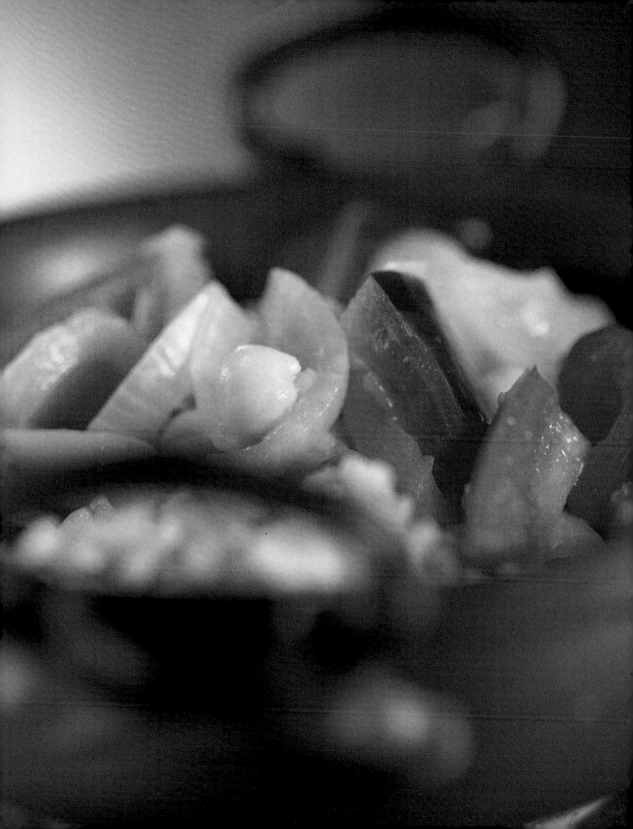

VEGETABLE PAELLA

Most people I meet are so deficient in B vitamins that it shocks me.
Low energy, weight issues, and many other niggly health complaints
often result. Enter rice to the rescue. Brown rice is loaded with
B vitamins and incredibly easy to prepare.

SERVES 4
½ cup long-grain brown rice
Sea salt
2 tsp olive oil
2 onions, peeled and diced
2 celery stalks, trimmed and thinly sliced
2 carrots, trimmed, peeled, and thinly sliced
6 cauliflower florets
½ tsp turmeric powder
Few strands of saffron
1 zucchini, trimmed and thinly sliced
Half a red pepper, seeded and thinly sliced
2 ounces fresh garden peas
2 tbsp chopped fresh parsley

1. Place the rice in a medium saucepan with 1 cup slightly salted water.
Bring to a boil, then lower the heat and simmer for 20–25 minutes, until
the liquid is absorbed. The rice should be cooked but slightly firm.
Remove from the heat and allow to stand for 10 minutes.
2. Place the oil in a saucepan with a little water. Add the onions, celery, and
carrots and cook for a few minutes to soften but not color the vegetables.
3. Add the cauliflower, turmeric, and saffron and cook for 5 minutes. Add the
zucchini and pepper, cook for an additional 2 minutes, then stir in the rice.
Sprinkle over the peas and parsley and serve.

SHIITAKE MUSHROOM RISOTTO

Barley has a sweet flavor and is particularly good for indigestion, edema, or dry skin. It does contain gluten, a substance to which some people are sensitive, but in very low levels.

SERVES 4
2 tbsp olive oil
1 large onion, peeled and chopped
2 garlic cloves, peeled and finely chopped
1 cup pearl barley, rinsed and drained
1 wheat-free vegetable stock cube
¼ pound shiitake mushrooms, trimmed and thinly sliced
2 tbsp chopped fresh parsley

1. Heat 1 tablespoon of olive oil and 1 tablespoon of water in a medium pan. Add the onion and garlic and cook over low heat until soft but not colored.

2. Stir in the barley, add 1.5 cups cold water, and the stock cube. Bring to a boil, then lower the heat and allow to simmer for about 10 minutes, until the barley is tender and all the liquid has been absorbed.

3. Heat the remaining olive oil in a small pan and sauté the mushrooms for 2–3 minutes. Stir into the risotto mixture with the freshly chopped parsley and serve.

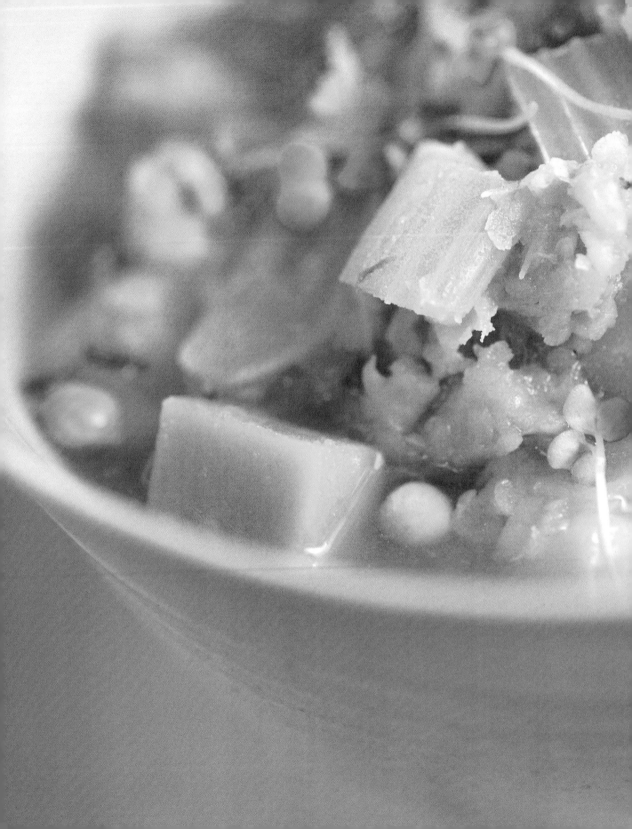

HEARTY LENTIL STEW

This dish is a superb way to strengthen the nervous system. When stressed, the kidneys take a beating and the adrenals pump out too many stress hormones, depleting the body of much-needed vitamin B. It's also a good transitional dish, as it contains a few white potatoes. If you're on a weight-loss program, then simply leave them out.

The key to maintaining the flavor of this is not to overcook the lentils. You'll know this has happened if they start to break up.

SERVES 4
½ **pound brown lentils**
2 onions, peeled and finely chopped
1 wheat-free vegetable stock cube
4 carrots, trimmed, peeled, and chopped
Half a butternut squash, peeled, seeded, and chopped
1 sweet potato, peeled and diced
4 small white potatoes, peeled and diced
1 celery stalk, trimmed and chopped
2 ounces fresh garden peas
¼ **pound fresh watercress**
2 tbsp chopped fresh dill
1 tsp tamari sauce

1. Soak the lentils in cold water for 20 minutes. Rinse thoroughly and drain.
2. Place the onions and vegetable stock cube in a saucepan with 3 cups water and bring to a boil. Add the lentils, carrots, squash, sweet potato, and white potatoes. Bring back to a boil, then lower the heat and simmer for 10 minutes. Add the celery and simmer for an additional 5 minutes.
3. Add the peas, watercress, dill, and tamari and serve with salt-free sauerkraut.

To turn this into a soup for the next day, add more water, extra fresh herbs of your choice, and some more stock and blend until smooth. Fabulous.

MUSHROOM STROGANOFF

My favorite mushrooms are shiitake, for their immune system boosting properties. If you suffer from thrush or yeast conditions, then stay away from mushrooms, with the exception of shiitakes.

SERVES 4
1 red onion, peeled and thinly sliced
2 tsp olive oil
1 garlic clove, peeled and finely chopped
¼ pound shiitake mushrooms, trimmed
4 large portobello mushrooms, trimmed and thickly sliced
¼ pound cremini mushrooms, some sliced, some whole
½ cup soy milk
3 tbsp chopped fresh flat-leaf parsley

1. Place the onion in a medium skillet with the olive oil and 1 tablespoon of water and cook gently for 2–3 minutes. Add the garlic and mushrooms and cook for an additional 3–4 minutes.
2. Add the soy milk and cook for an additional 5 minutes over medium heat. Sprinkle on the parsley and serve with Gourmet Brown Rice (see page 195).

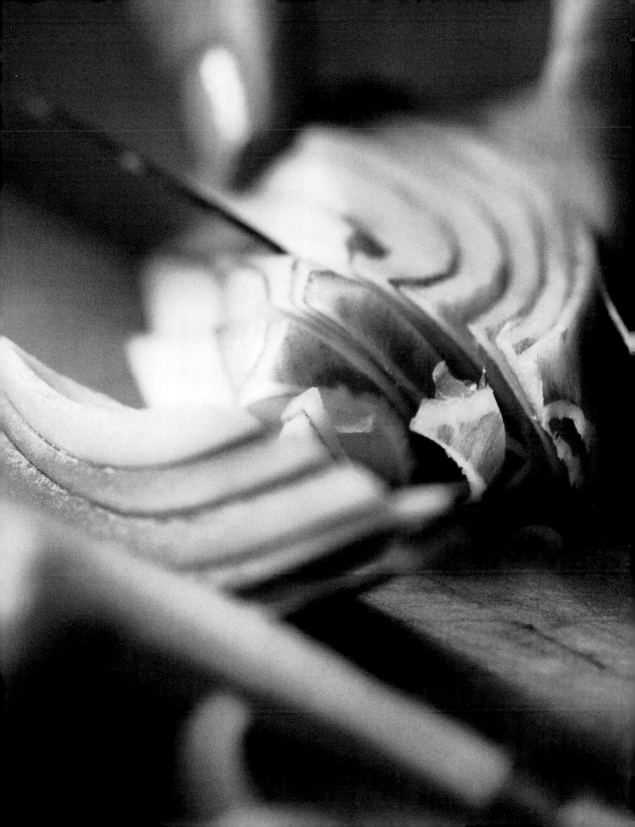

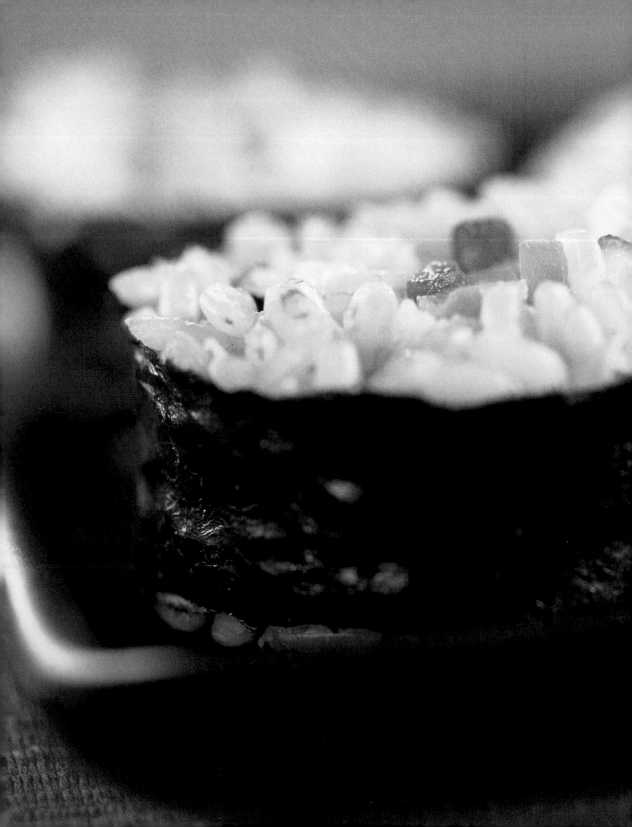

VEGETABLE SUSHI ROLLS

This is one of the best dishes to get your children involved in the kitchen. Children eating seaweed? They love it. In fact, nori is my favorite sea veggie because of its high nutrient vitamin and mineral content. Nori is also a great source of protein and the most easily digested of all the sea vegetables. If you are prone to colds, have high blood pressure, catarrh, water retention, or lack of energy, this is your dish.

SERVES 4–6

1 cup brown rice
1 wheat-free vegetable stock cube
½ ounce nori sushi sheets (1 nori sheet for each person)
2 avocados, flesh mashed with a squeeze of lime or lemon juice
Half a cucumber, peeled and cut into julienne (matchstick) strips
Half a small white cabbage, shredded

1 large carrot, trimmed, peeled, and grated
3 ounces alfalfa sprouts
1 small red onion, peeled and finely chopped
1 red pepper, seeded and finely shredded
1 tbsp pickled ginger or sushi daikon

1. Place the rice and stock cube in a small saucepan and add 2 cups of boiling water. Bring back to a boil, cover, lower the heat, and simmer for 7–10 minutes, or until the water has been absorbed. Remove from the heat and cool.
2. Place a sushi sheet on a flat surface or on a bamboo mat, if you have one. Spread evenly with the mashed avocado, leaving 1 inch of the sheet uncovered at the far end. Spread with a thin layer of rice.
3. Arrange a row of each remaining ingredient in the center of the roll. Carefully fold the edge of the sheet closest to you over the filling. Tuck the end in and begin to roll, as tightly as possible. Before you reach the end, moisten the top edge of the nori sheet with a little water so that it sticks. Wrap in plastic and place in the fridge until ready to serve.
4. Repeat with the remaining sheets.
5. To serve, slice the sushi with a very sharp knife into 1-inch pieces. Serve with a little tamari sauce to dip.

TOP TIP

Don't make the nori rolls too thick—they need to be eaten in one bite. Find the ideal proportions. But if you are involving the kids, let them have fun—that's the whole point of this dish! Eventually, you will become an expert sushi roller, and so will your kids.

TEMPEH AUTUMN STEW

Tempeh is compressed soybeans and can be bought in a health food store fresh, frozen, or precooked. It's an excellent meat substitute, is high in omega 3 "good" fats and the energy vitamin, B_{12}. I use pumpkin in this dish, as it's helpful for regulating blood sugar levels. If you have diabetes, suffer from hypoglycemia (blood sugar swings), or get shaky if you don't eat at regular intervals, then this dish could help.

SERVES 4
6–9 whole pearl onions, peeled
2 tbsp olive oil
8-ounce block tempeh
1 strip kombu sea vegetable
3 carrots, trimmed, peeled, and cut into chunks
1-inch piece fresh ginger, peeled and sliced
2 sprigs fresh rosemary
1 tbsp wheat-free vegetable bouillon powder
4 sprigs fresh thyme
Quarter of a small pumpkin, peeled and cut into large pieces
¼ pound fresh garden peas
2 tsp mugi miso
2 tbsp chopped fresh parsley

1. Place the onions and oil in a medium casserole dish. Add enough water to cover them and boil for 2–3 minutes.
2. Add the tempeh, kombu, carrots, ginger, rosemary, bouillon powder, and thyme. Add more water to cover the vegetables. Cover and bring to a boil, then lower the heat and simmer uncovered for 10 minutes.
3. Add the pumpkin and simmer for an addtional 10 minutes.
4. Blanch the peas in boiling water for 2–3 minutes. Drain and refresh in cold water.
5. Take 2 tablespoons of juice from the casserole dish and mix with the mugi miso and return to the pan. Serve with the peas and garnished with the parsley.

TEMPEH WITH SWEET AND SOUR RED CABBAGE

Cabbage strengthens the liver and contains anti-cancer nutrients, so don't skimp on it. I use the seaweed kombu to enhance the flavor of the tempeh and also as a tenderizer. I often use it in bean dishes too, as it helps to remove the substances which cause gas.

SERVES 4

8-ounce block tempeh
1 strip kombu sea vegetable
2 tsp tamari sauce
4 onions, peeled and thinly sliced
2 bay leaves
Half a red cabbage, finely shredded
sea salt
1 tsp allspice

$\frac{1}{2}$ tsp freshly grated nutmeg
3 tbsp rice vinegar
3 tbsp freshly pressed apple juice
1 tbsp olive oil
2 tsp arrowroot dissolved
in 1 tbsp cold water
2 spring onions, trimmed and thinly sliced
2 carrots, trimmed, peeled, and finely grated

1. Cut the tempeh into 4 pieces and place in a medium pan with the kombu and tamari. Half-cover the tempeh with water and bring to a boil. Lower the heat and simmer for 10 minutes, then drain. Discard the kombu.

2. Place the onions in a medium casserole dish and add enough water to cover. Add the bay leaves, bring to a boil, then lower the heat and simmer for 5–7 minutes. Add the cabbage, seasonings, vinegar, and apple juice and cook for an addtional 10–15 minutes.

3. Heat the oil in a small skillet with 2 tablespoons of water, add the tempeh, and pan-fry for a couple of minutes on each side.

4. Add the arrowroot to the red cabbage mixture.

5. Put the tempeh on top of the cabbage and serve garnished with the spring onions and grated carrot.

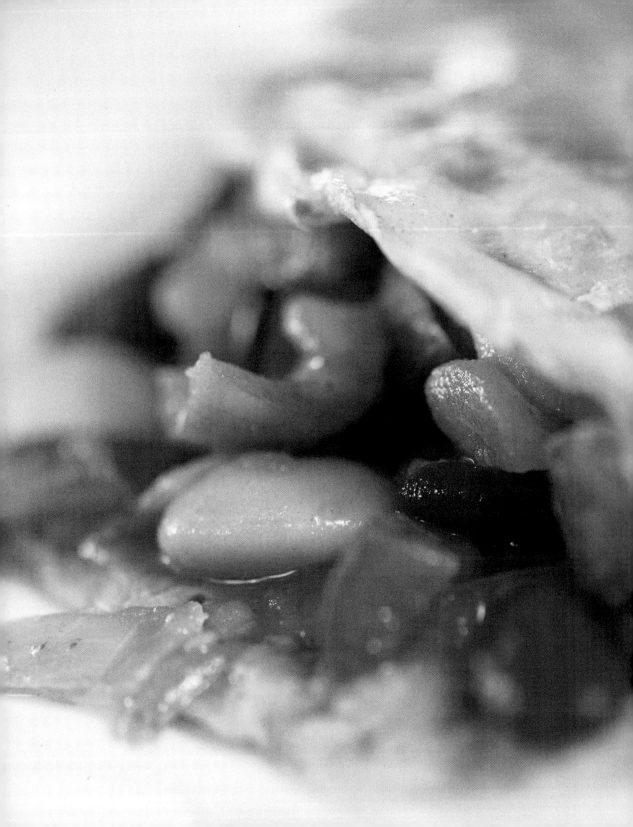

WHOLE-WHEAT OAT PANCAKES WITH RATATOUILLE

Oats are soothing to the body's nervous system, strengthening to the stomach and spleen, and good cholesterol-busters. They have also been found to be a good friend to the sex drive. You have probably heard of the saying "sow your wild oats." So you can do that with my pancakes. Sometimes I also add raw sprouted seeds to the filling.

SERVES 4–6

Pancakes:
1 cup whole-wheat flour
2 tbsp oat bran
Avocado oil or virgin olive oil
Filling:
1 small onion, peeled and finely chopped
1 garlic clove, peeled and finely chopped
1 red pepper, seeded and finely chopped
1 yellow or green pepper, seeded and finely chopped

16-ounce can chopped organic tomatoes
1 eggplant, trimmed and chopped into 1-inch pieces (optional)
2 zucchinis, trimmed, halved lengthwise, and sliced
1 tbsp wheat-free vegetable bouillon powder
16-ounce can no salt mixed beans
4–6 sprigs fresh basil

1. Blend the flour and oat bran together with 1 cup cold water in a food processor or with a handheld blender for 1 minute. Allow to rest while you prepare the filling.
2. Place the onion, garlic, peppers, tomatoes, eggplant, and zucchini in a medium pan with the bouillon powder and 1 tablespoon of hot water.
3. Cook over medium heat for 10–15 minutes, then stir in the beans. Cook for an addtional 5 minutes. Remove from the heat and set aside.
4. Heat an 8-inch nonstick skillet, drizzle with a little oil, and then wipe with a piece of paper towel. Add a thin layer of batter to coat the base of the pan; tilt the pan to coat evenly.
5. Cook for 2 minutes, or until the sides of the pancake begin to lift. Slide a palette knife underneath and flip the pancake carefully onto the other side. Cook for an additional 2 minutes, or until set and lightly browned.
6. Slide the pancake onto a plate and keep warm in the oven. Repeat with the remaining mixture. Reheat the filling and spoon into the center of the prepared pancakes. Fold over the pancakes and place on warmed serving plates. Garnish with the basil sprigs.

ROOT VEGETABLES AND
TOFU EN PAPILLOTE

Tofu is a very good source of protein. Researchers have discovered that regular intake of soy protein can help lower too-high cholesterol levels. Tofu also contains phytoestrogens, which have been shown to alleviate symptoms associated with menopause. Tofu tends to be neutral in taste and will take on the flavor of the seasonings in a dish.

SERVES 4
2 tsp olive oil
2 carrots, trimmed, peeled, and cut into fine julienne (matchstick) strips
1 parsnip, trimmed, peeled, and cut into fine julienne (matchstick) strips
2 sweet potatoes, peeled and cut into fine julienne (matchstick) strips
2 zucchinis, trimmed and cut into fine julienne (matchstick) strips
8-ounce block smoked tofu, cut into 1-inch cubes
1 tsp ground cumin
2 tsp tamari sauce
4 tsp freshly pressed apple juice
4 bay leaves
2 tbsp sesame seeds
¼ cup fresh bean sprouts

1. Preheat the oven to 400°F.
2. Take 4 pieces of foil, 12 inches square, and brush the center of each with a little oil.
3. Mix all the vegetables together in a large bowl and divide among the foil sheets.
4. Place the tofu on top of the vegetables. Season with the cumin and bring the foil up around the vegetables to form a parcel. Add the tamari and apple juice and top with a bay leaf. Add a little water to each parcel and then scrunch up the foil to seal everything in.
5. Transfer to the oven and bake for 20 minutes.
6. Remove from the oven and allow to stand for 5 minutes. Transfer the foil parcels to serving plates. Open up the parcels slightly and sprinkle on the sesame seeds and sprouts and serve immediately.

TOFU WITH STEAMED VEGETABLES

SERVES 4
2 zucchinis, trimmed and sliced
3 carrots, trimmed, peeled, and sliced
¼ pound green beans, trimmed
1 head broccoli, cut into florets
1 tbsp olive oil
1 garlic clove, peeled and crushed
1 tsp tamari sauce
2 tbsp freshly pressed apple juice
8-ounce block smoked tofu, cut into 1-inch cubes
Fresh basil and parsley

1. Steam the vegetables one at a time in an electric steamer or over a pan of boiling water. Steam the zucchini first for 3–4 minutes and then the carrots for 7–8 minutes.
2. Blanch the beans and broccoli in boiling water for 3–4 minutes, drain well, and refresh in cold water.
3. Heat the oil in a medium casserole pan with 1 tablespoon of water, then add the garlic and cook for 1 minute. Add all the cooked vegetables, the tamari, apple juice, tofu, and herbs and cook for 1 minute. Serve immediately.

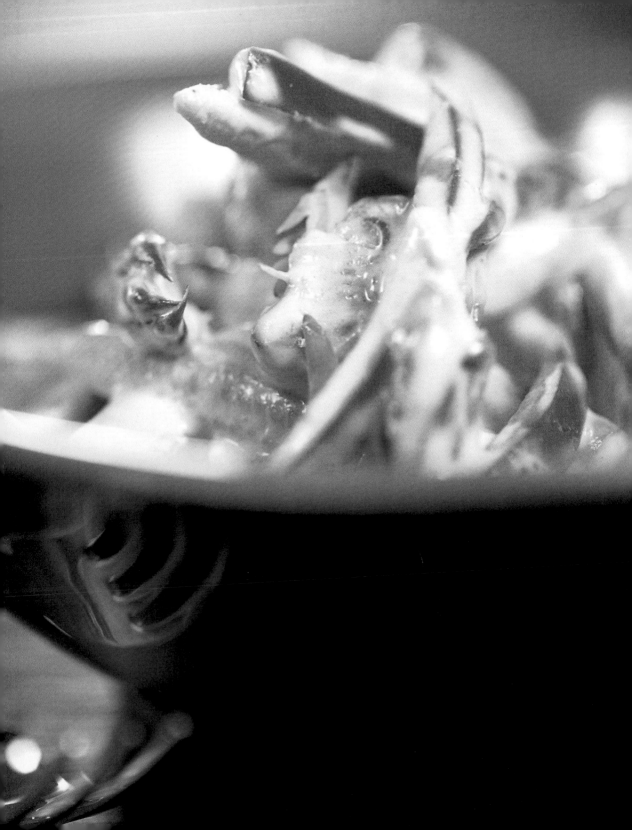

FRAGRANT THAI VEGETABLE CURRY

SERVES 4–6
15-ounce can coconut milk
½ tsp ground coriander
½ tsp ground cumin
2 kaffir lime leaves
1-inch piece fresh ginger, peeled and sliced
2 stalks lemongrass, cut into 1-inch pieces
2 tbsp chopped fresh cilantro
¼ pound snap peas
Half a red pepper, seeded and diced
Half a yellow pepper, seeded and diced
¼ pound baby corn, halved lengthwise
1 eggplant, trimmed and chopped
2 zucchinis, trimmed and chopped
2 spring onions, trimmed and thinly sliced
1 handful of bean sprouts
A few fresh basil leaves to garnish

1. Heat the coconut milk in a wok until boiling, then add the spices, lime leaves, ginger, lemongrass, and cilantro. Cook for 2–3 minutes over high heat.
2. Add the peas, peppers, baby corn, eggplant, and zucchini and cook for an addtional 3–4 minutes, or until the vegetables are just cooked.
3. Sprinkle on the spring onions, bean sprouts, and basil and serve immediately from the wok with brown rice.

VEGETARIAN CHILI

SERVES 4

Two 16-ounce cans kidney beans, drained and rinsed
11-ounce can corn, drained and rinsed
Two 16-ounce cans chopped organic tomatoes
1 onion, peeled and cut into large chunks
2 zucchinis, trimmed and diced
¼ pound frozen fava beans
1 garlic clove, peeled and chopped
2 tsp ground cardamom
2 tsp ground cinnamon
1 tbsp tamari sauce
1 tbsp chopped fresh basil
1 handful bean sprouts
1 large beefsteak tomato, roughly chopped
1 spring onion, trimmed and chopped

1. Preheat the oven to 350°F.
2. Mix all the ingredients except the spring onion together in a large bowl. Transfer to a large casserole dish and bake for 35–40 minutes.
3. Remove from the oven and serve garnished with the bean sprouts and spring onion. Serve with brown rice.

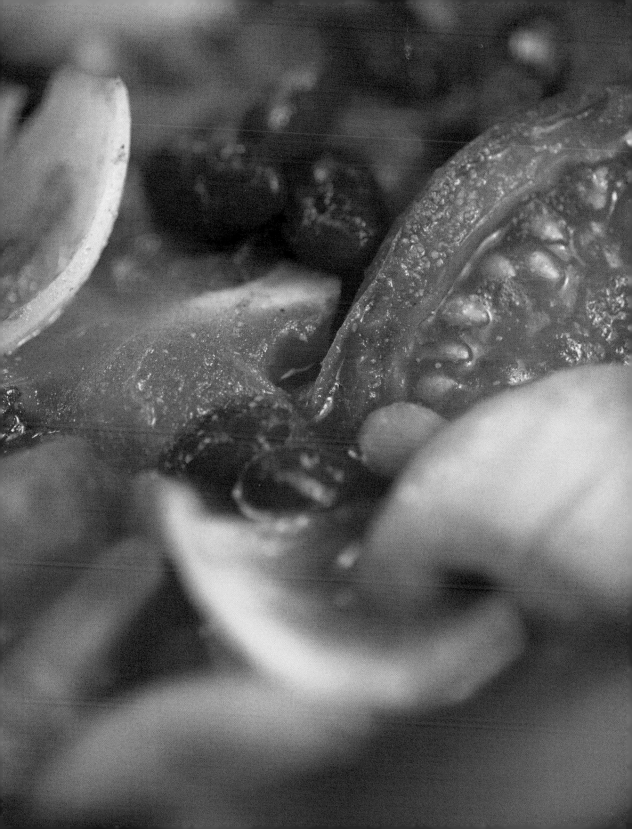

CHICKPEA AND TOFU MILD CURRY

SERVES 4
1 tbsp olive oil
3 onions, peeled and diced
Sea salt
Half a 16-ounce block fresh tofu, cut into 1-inch cubes
16-ounce can chickpeas, drained and rinsed
2 tbsp chopped fresh cilantro
2 carrots, trimmed, peeled, and diced
1 tsp ground cumin
1 tsp ground turmeric
1 tsp ground coriander
1 tbsp mugi miso
1 tbsp arrowroot dissolved in 1 tbsp water
1 pound kale or collard greens, tough stems removed and roughly shredded
Fresh cilantro leaves, to garnish

1. Heat the oil in a medium pan and add the onions and a pinch
of salt. Cook gently for 10 minutes, until soft and translucent.
2. Add the tofu, chickpeas, cilantro, carrots, spices, and enough water
to cover. Bring to a boil, lower the heat, cover, and cook for 10 minutes.
3. Take 2 tablespoons of the cooking juices and mix with the mugi
miso and add to the stew along with the arrowroot mixture.
4. Bring a large pan of water to a boil and cook the kale or collard greens
for 3–4 minutes.
5. Strain and arrange on warmed serving plates. Top with the curry,
garnish with cilantro leaves, and serve immediately.

MUNG BEAN CASSEROLE

This is the best dish for ridding the body of toxins and bacteria.

SERVES 4
$\frac{1}{2}$ pound mung beans, soaked for 6 hours in cold water
1 wheat-free vegetable stock cube
$1\frac{1}{2}$ tsp turmeric powder
$1\frac{1}{2}$ tsp ground cumin
3 tbsp chopped fresh cilantro
1 onion, peeled and finely chopped
2 carrots, trimmed, peeled, and chopped
2 endives, leaves separated
1 small bunch radishes, trimmed and halved
A few clover sprouts

1. Drain the mung beans and rinse well.
2. Bring 3 cups water to a boil and add the mung beans, stock cube, turmeric, and cumin; lower the heat and simmer for 30 minutes. Then add the cilantro, onion, and carrots and simmer for a few more minutes.
3. Arrange the endive around the edge of a deep bowl, spoon in the casserole mixture, and garnish with the radishes and clover sprouts. Serve with brown rice and a hearty salad.

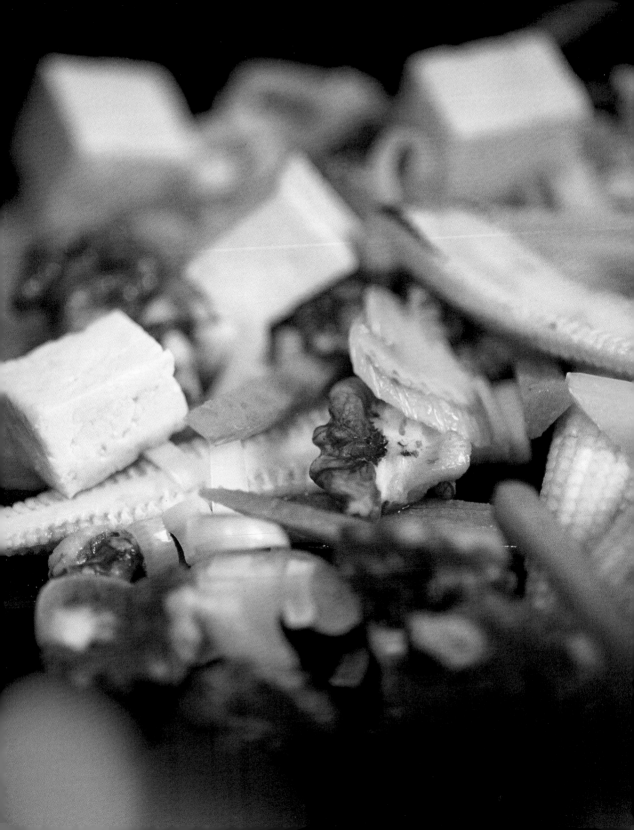

TOFU PECAN STIR-FRY

SERVES 4

2 leeks, washed, trimmed, and thinly sliced
1 tsp tamari sauce
2 carrots, trimmed, peeled, and cut
into fine julienne (matchstick) strips
8-ounce block smoked tofu, cut into
1-inch cubes

4 ounces baby corn, halved lengthwise
3 celery stalks, trimmed and sliced
3–4 tbsp chopped pecans
1 tsp sesame oil
1 tsp grated orange rind

1. Heat a large wok, add a little water, and then the leeks and tamari.
Stir-fry for a few minutes, and then add the carrots, tofu, and baby corn.
Cook for an additional 5 minutes.
2. Add the celery, pecans, sesame oil, and orange rind. Serve immediately
on a bed of salad leaves.

AROMATIC POACHED CHICKEN

SERVES 4

4 skinless organic chicken breasts
1 wheat-free vegetable stock cube
1 stalk lemongrass, cut into 1-inch pieces
2 kaffir lime leaves
1-inch piece fresh ginger, peeled and
thinly sliced

2 celery stalks, trimmed and sliced
1 leek, washed, trimmed, and thinly sliced
¼ pound shiitake mushrooms
1 bunch watercress, trimmed
¼ pound bean sprouts
3 tbsp chopped fresh cilantro

1. Place the chicken breasts in a medium pan of water with the
stock cube, lemongrass, lime leaves, and ginger and bring to a boil.
2. Add the celery and leek, lower the heat, and simmer for 20 minutes.
3. Add the mushrooms and cook for an additional 2 minutes.
4. Remove from the heat. Take out the chicken breast and diagonally slice.
5. Add the watercress, bean sprouts, and cilantro to the pan.
6. Divide among 4 soup bowls, top with the sliced chicken breast, and serve.

CHAPTER 9

QUICK BITES

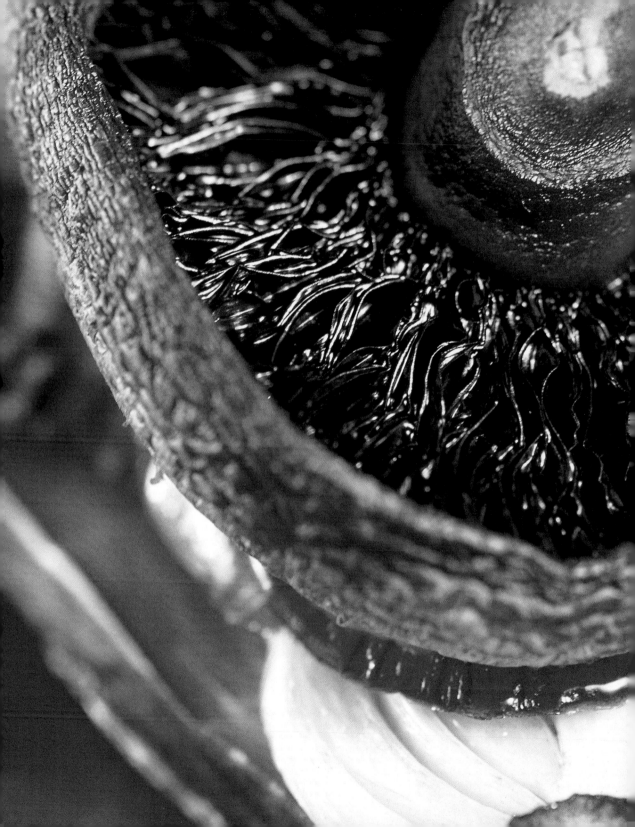

TOO BUSY TO EAT HEALTHFULLY? I HEAR THIS ALL THE TIME, BUT I URGE YOU NOT TO FALL INTO THE TRAP OF THE QUICK-FIX, BOIL IN THE BAG, PROCESSED, JUNK FOOD LIFESTYLE. "CONVENIENCE" IS A MISNOMER FOR THESE FOODS. IT'S NOT SO CONVENIENT TO FEEL TIRED OR UNWELL, LIVE WITH HEADACHES, BLOATING, GAS, OR WEIGHT PROBLEMS. ALL RISE FOR MY EXTRA QUICK BITES. THESE MEALS WERE BORN OUT OF A CHALLENGE, AND I ALWAYS LIKE A CHALLENGE. ONE OF THE PARTICIPANTS ON THE TV PROGRAM *YOU ARE WHAT YOU EAT* CHALLENGED ME TO SHOW HER MEALS THAT COULD BE PREPARED IN THE TIME THAT SHE WOULD OPEN HER FROZEN DINNERS AND HEAT THEM UP. REMEMBER SMOOTHIES ONLY TAKE ABOUT THREE MINUTES TO PREPARE, SO BREAKFAST WAS EASY. AND THROWING TOGETHER A SALAD IS REALLY QUICK. HOT DISHES WERE MORE OF A CHALLENGE, BUT I STARTED OFF WITH THIS SIMPLE POACHED CHICKEN WITH VEGGIES, AND THINGS SOON DEVELOPED FROM THERE. IF YOU ARE ON A WEIGHT-LOSS PROGRAM, OR SUFFER FROM BLOATING, THEN AVOID THE PASTA RECIPES.

POACHED CHICKEN WITH VEGETABLES

SERVES 2

1 organic skinless chicken breast

1 tsp organic wheat-free vegetable bouillon powder

2 carrots, trimmed, peeled, and sliced

1 leek, washed, trimmed, and sliced

2 ounces fresh or frozen peas

1 tsp cornstarch

1 tsp chopped fresh parsley

1. Cut the chicken breast into chunks and place in a saucepan with 2 cups water and the vegetable bouillon powder. Add the carrots and leek and bring to a boil. Lower the heat and simmer for 5 minutes, then add the peas. Return to a boil and simmer for 2 more minutes, until the chicken is cooked.

2. Blend the cornstarch with 1 tablespoon of cold water and stir into the chicken mixture. Cook for a few seconds, until the cooking liquid has thickened.

3. Stir through the chopped parsley and serve immediately with lightly cooked cabbage.

GRILLED EGGPLANT AND MUSHROOM STACK

SERVES 4

1 large eggplant, trimmed and cut lengthwise into ¾-inch slices
1 fennel bulb, trimmed and sliced
1 red onion, peeled and thinly sliced
4 large flat mushrooms, trimmed
1 tbsp olive oil
4 garlic cloves, peeled and chopped

1. Preheat the oven to 400°F.
2. Arrange the vegetables on a large baking sheet and glaze the eggplant, fennel slices, and onion with olive oil using a pastry brush.
3. Scatter the garlic over the vegetables.
4. Bake for 8–10 minutes, or until lightly colored.
5. Arrange the eggplant on 4 warm serving plates, top with the fennel, then the onion, and finally the whole mushrooms. Serve immediately with a green salad.

BBQ FISH KEBABS

SERVES 2
Sauce:
1 red pepper, halved and seeded
4 tomatoes, halved
2 tsp olive oil
1 tsp paprika
2 tbsp chopped fresh basil

$3/4$ pound firm white fish such as monkfish,
cut into chunks
1 red onion, peeled and quartered
4 cherry tomatoes
1 yellow pepper, seeded and cut into
$1\frac{1}{2}$-inch squares
1 zucchini, trimmed and cut into chunks

1. Fire up the grill. If not using a barbecue, preheat the oven to 400°F.
2. To make the sauce, place the peppers and tomatoes on a baking sheet, cut
side up, drizzle with the olive oil, and roast for 10 minutes. Allow to cool
slightly, then place in a food processor. Add the paprika and basil and
blend until smooth. Transfer to a serving bowl.
3. Thread the fish alternately with the vegetables onto 4 large skewers.
Cook for 3–4 minutes each side on the grill or bake in the oven for 7–10
minutes. Serve immediately with the sauce on the side.

STUFFED ZUCCHINI

SERVES 2
2 large zucchinis, halved lengthwise
and flesh removed with a teaspoon
8 cherry tomatoes, halved
12 black pitted olives
4 ounces goat cheese, crumbled
1 tsp olive oil
12 fresh basil leaves, roughly torn

1. Preheat the oven to 400°F.
2. Line a baking with aluminum foil and place the zucchini boats on the foil. Arrange the cherry tomatoes, olives, and goat cheese alternately in the zucchinis. Drizzle with a little olive oil, and sprinkle over half the basil leaves.
3. Bake for 20 minutes and serve immediately, garnished with the rest of the basil leaves.

PASTA WITH ROASTED CHERRY TOMATOES

I am not an advocate of eating pasta every single day. Make it once in a while and try out green pastas and wheat-free variations.

SERVES 2

½ cup pine nuts
½ pound wheat-free pasta
8 ounces cherry tomatoes, halved
2 tsp olive oil

¼ cup chopped fresh basil
Balsamic vinegar to dress

1. Preheat the oven to 400°F.
2. Place the pine nuts in a small pan over low heat and toast, stirring frequently until golden in color. Set aside.
3. Bring a medium pan of water to a boil, add the pasta, and cook for 3–4 minutes, or until al dente.
4. Meanwhile, place the cherry tomatoes on a baking sheet and drizzle with a little olive oil. Roast for 4–5 minutes.
5. Drain the pasta, then toss with the tomatoes and their juices, the basil, and toasted pine nuts. Drizzle with balsamic vinegar and serve.

GRILLED PEPPERS WITH CANNELLINI BEANS AND BLACK OLIVES

SERVES 2

4 mixed peppers, halved and seeded
Olive oil, to brush
16-ounce can cannellini beans, drained
and rinsed
¼ chopped black olives

1 garlic clove, peeled and chopped
2 tbsp chopped fresh parsley
2 tsp olive oil

1. Brush the skin side of the peppers with olive oil. Heat a grill pan until very hot, then place the peppers skin side down on the pan. Cook until the skin is beginning to wrinkle, then remove from the heat and allow to cool.
2. Place the beans, olives, garlic, and parsley in a medium bowl. Add the olive oil and mix well.
3. Cut the peppers into thick slices, add to the beans, and serve.

PASTA SALAD

SERVES 2

¼ pound wheat-free pasta
1 zucchini, trimmed and cut into julienne (matchstick) strips
1 red pepper, seeded and thinly sliced
1 yellow pepper, seeded and thinly sliced
1 ounce canned corn, drained and rinsed
2 spring onions, trimmed and finely chopped
2 tbsp chopped fresh dill
2 tbsp capers (optional)
Sesame Miso Dressing (see page 228)

1. Bring a medium pan of water to a boil, add the pasta, and cook for 2–3 minutes, or until al dente (just cooked). Drain and refresh in cold water. Drain well and place in a salad bowl.
2. Place a little water in a medium pan and cook the zucchini for 2–3 minutes. Add the peppers, mix well, and remove from the heat. Toss the zucchini and peppers into the cooked pasta along with all the other ingredients.
3. Just before serving, toss through some Sesame Miso Dressing.

BUCKWHEAT SALAD

SERVES 2

½ cup buckwheat groats
Half a red pepper, seeded and finely chopped
2 carrots, trimmed, peeled, and finely diced
2 onions, peeled and finely chopped
1 bay leaf
2 tbsp diced pickles
2 tsp chopped fresh dill
2 spring onions, trimmed and finely chopped
Dressing:
1 tbsp peanut butter
1 tbsp Dijon mustard
1 tsp white miso paste
1 tbsp freshly pressed apple juice

1. Rinse the buckwheat and drain. Place in a medium saucepan.
2. Add the pepper, carrots, onions, bay leaf, and enough water to cover.
3. Bring to a boil, then lower the heat and simmer for 15–20 minutes. All liquid should be reduced; drain if necessary.
4. Mix in the pickle, dill, and spring onions.
5. Mix the dressing ingredients with 2 tablespoons of hot water, drizzle over the salad, and serve.

QUICK TOFU

SERVES 2

1 tbsp olive oil	$\frac{1}{2}$ tsp turmeric powder
2 onions, peeled and finely chopped	Half a 16-ounce block tofu
2 ounces canned corn, drained and rinsed	Half an 8-ounce block smoked tofu
$\frac{1}{4}$ pound shiitake mushrooms, trimmed	1 bunch watercress
Juice of half a lemon	2 tbsp pine nuts

1. In a medium pan, heat the oil and the onion with 2 tablespoons of water. Cook for 10 minutes, until soft but not colored.
2. Add the corn, mushrooms, lemon juice, and turmeric and stir. Crumble in the tofu. Cook for an additional 10 minutes.
3. Mix in the watercress and pine nuts and serve.

GOURMET BROWN RICE

SERVES 1–2

$\frac{1}{2}$ cup brown rice
1 wheat-free vegetable stock cube or 2 tsp miso paste
2 carrots, trimmed, peeled, and thinly sliced
1 celery stalk, trimmed and thinly sliced

1. Place the rice in a small saucepan with 1 cup water and add the stock cube or miso and the vegetables.
2. Bring to a boil, then lower the heat and simmer for 20 minutes, until the rice is tender but not all the liquid is absorbed. Turn off the heat and allow to stand for 10 minutes before serving.

QUICK LENTIL STEW WITH ARTICHOKES

SERVES 2
½ **pound Puy lentils**
1 onion, peeled and sliced
4 celery stalks, trimmed and sliced
4 carrots, trimmed, peeled, and sliced
3 parsnips, trimmed, peeled, and sliced
16-ounce can artichoke hearts
1 leek, washed, trimmed, and sliced
1 wheat-free vegetable stock cube
¾ **pound kale leaves, chopped**
2 tbsp chopped fresh parsley or chervil

1. Rinse the Puy lentils and drain. Place in a large pan with all the other ingredients except the kale and herbs.
2. Add enough water to cover, bring to a boil, then lower the heat and simmer for 20 minutes.
3. Remove from the heat and mix in the kale leaves to warm through. Sprinkle on the herbs and serve.

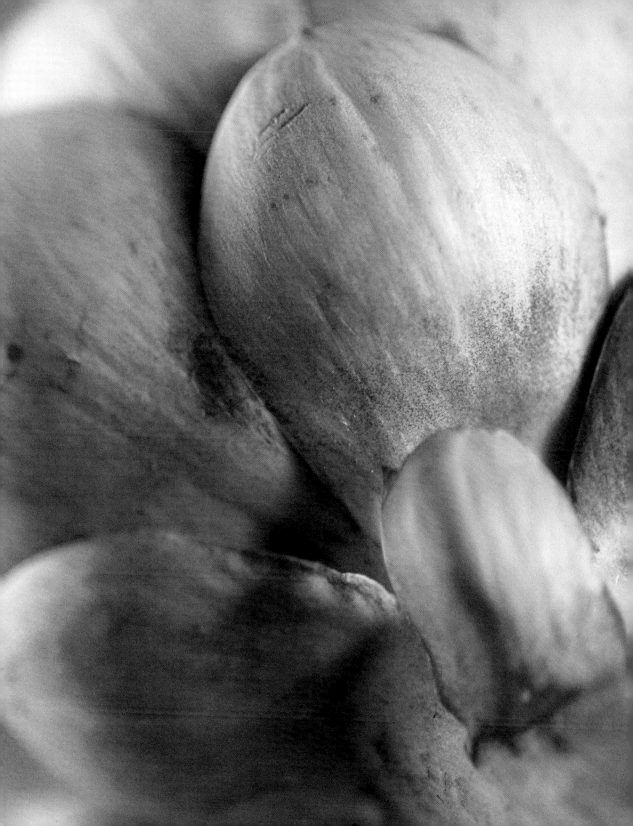

TUNA STEAKS WITH BLACK-EYED PEA SALSA

SERVES 2
Two 4-ounce tuna steaks
$^1/_2$ pound fresh arugula
$^1/_2$ pound fresh watercress
Salsa:
16-ounce can black-eyed peas, drained and rinsed
1 red onion, peeled and diced
1 red pepper, seeded and diced
1 beefsteak tomato, halved, seeded, and finely chopped
2 tbsp chopped fresh cilantro
2 tsp olive oil or hemp oil

1. Heat a grill pan until very hot. Sear the tuna for 2 minutes, then turn and cook the other side for 2–3 minutes. Remove from the heat and allow to cool.
2. To make the salsa, mix together the peas with the onion, pepper, tomato, cilantro, and oil.
3. Arrange the arugula and watercress on a plate.
4. Place the tuna on the salad, spoon the salsa over the top, and serve immediately.

STIR-FRIED VEGETABLES WITH ARAME

Don't be put off by the brown, stringy appearance of the seaweed arame. Arame is a source of calcium and iron. It is supportive for the spleen, pancreas, and stomach and is delicious in this recipe.

SERVES 2
2 ounces arame sea vegetable
10 pieces baby corn
1 onion, peeled and sliced
2 tsp olive oil
2 carrots, trimmed, peeled, and cut into julienne (matchstick) strips
1 bunch asparagus, cut into bite-size pieces
1 red pepper, seeded and thinly sliced
1 fennel bulb, trimmed, cored, and thinly sliced
Zest of half a lemon
$\frac{1}{2}$-inch piece ginger, peeled and grated
1 tbsp chopped fresh cilantro
1 tbsp chopped fresh chervil

1. Soak the arame in cold water for 10 minutes and drain well. Blanch the corn in boiling water for 2–3 minutes. Drain and refresh in cold water.
2. Place the onion, olive oil, and 2 tablespoons of water in a wok and cook for 5–7 minutes, until soft.
3. Add the arame, corn, and all the other ingredients except the cilantro and chervil, and cook for 2–3 minutes. Serve immediately, garnished with the cilantro and chervil.

CHAPTER 10

SNACKS

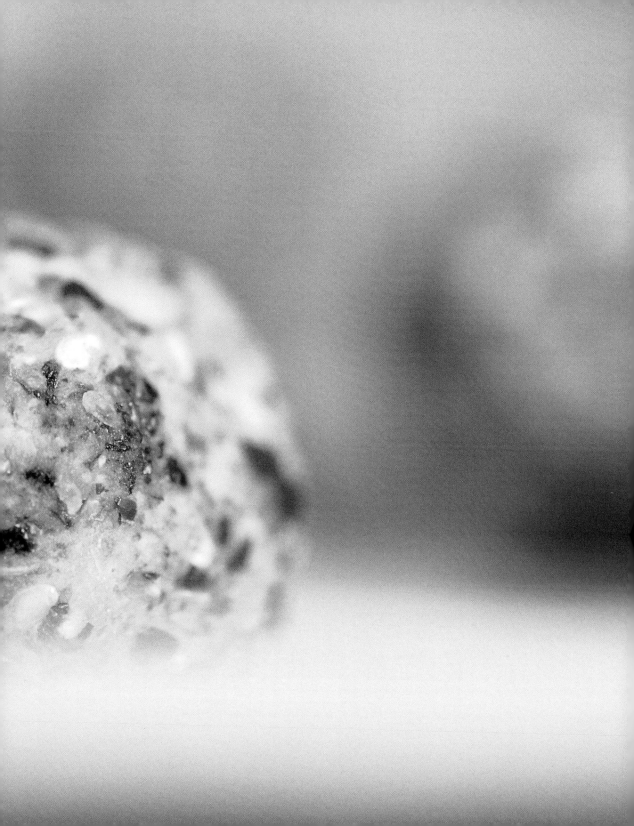

I WANT YOU TO CHANGE YOUR ENTIRE CONSCIOUSNESS ABOUT SNACKING. FROM THIS DAY FORWARD, YOUR MENTAL ASSOCIATION WITH THE WORD "SNACK" WILL BE TRANSFORMED. YOU WILL NO LONGER ASSOCIATE THE WORD "SNACK" WITH JUNK FOODS LIKE CHIPS, COOKIES, ICE CREAM, CAKES, AND CANDY. WHEN YOU NOW HEAR THE WORD "SNACK," YOU WILL THINK OF HEALTHY WHOLESOME GOODIES, SIMPLE YET AMAZING FOODS SUCH AS VEGETABLE STICKS, FRUITS, RAW NUTS, HEMP SEEDS, SUNFLOWER SEEDS, AND A WHOLE HOST OF OTHERS. YOU CAN MAKE THE LEAP. I DID IT YEARS AGO, AND I WOULD NOT EXPECT YOU TO DO SOMETHING THAT I HAVEN'T DONE MYSELF. IT WILL MAKE A HUGE DIFFERENCE TO YOUR LIFE.

CRUNCHY KALE

This can be eaten as a snack or sprinkled over pasta, risotto, or salads.

SERVES 4
Olive oil
¼ pound curly kale, stems removed
1 tsp dried mixed herbs

1. Preheat the oven to 350°F. Line a baking sheet with foil and lightly brush with a little olive oil using a pastry brush.
2. Cut the leaves into wide slices and arrange evenly spaced on the baking sheet.
3. Bake for 15–20 minutes, being sure to stir them at least twice while they're baking. The kale leaves are ready when they're bright green and crisp.
4. Remove the leaves from the oven and season with dried mixed herbs. Eat on the same day.

SESAME RICE BALLS

This is also delicious served cold. Umeboshi is an easy-to-digest vegetable protein snack. It has an alkalizing effect on the body, which is good for people who have eaten excess amounts of red meat (one too many burgers and fries!).

MAKES ABOUT 12
1 cup brown rice
½ cup sesame seeds
16-ounce can kidney beans, drained and rinsed
2 tsp umeboshi paste
¼ cup lemon juice
Tamari sauce, for dipping

1. Preheat the oven to 350°F. Line a baking sheet with parchment paper.
2. Bring a large pan of water to a boil. Add the rice and cook for 20 minutes. Drain and rinse in cold water.
3. Heat the sesame seeds in a medium pan over medium heat until lightly toasted.
4. Place the rice, beans, umeboshi paste, and lemon juice in a food processor and process until it forms a stiff mixture.
5. Roll the rice mixture into walnut-size balls, then roll in the sesame seeds and place on the prepared baking sheet.
6. Bake for 12–15 minutes, until hot, and serve with the tamari as a dipping sauce.

My spreads are
very versatile. Add
to salads for extra
flavor; use as dips
for veggie crudités
and spread on my
Squash Bread
(see page 212) for a
delicious snack any
time of the day.

SESAME SQUASH SPREAD

MAKES ABOUT ½ CUP
KEEPS FOR TWO DAYS IN THE FRIDGE OR ONE MONTH IN THE FREEZER
1 pound butternut squash, peeled, seeded, and cut into 1-inch pieces
5 tbsp sesame seeds
1 tsp brown miso paste
1 pinch cinnamon

1. Place the squash in a medium saucepan and cover with water.
Bring to a boil, then lower the heat and simmer for 10–15 minutes, until
tender when pierced with a knife. Drain well and blend in a food processor
or with a handheld blender.
2. Heat the sesame seeds in a small pan until lightly toasted and add
to the purée with the miso and cinnamon.
3. Blend until smooth, adding a little water if necessary.
4. Transfer to a small bowl and cover. Place in the fridge until ready to use.

GINGER SQUASH BUTTER

MAKES ABOUT ½ CUP
KEEPS FOR TWO DAYS IN THE FRIDGE OR ONE MONTH IN THE FREEZER
1 pound butternut squash, peeled, seeded, and cut into 1-inch pieces
1 tbsp miso paste
1-inch piece fresh ginger, finely grated
Zest of half a lemon

1. Place the squash in a medium pan and cover with cold water.
2. Bring to a boil, then lower the heat and simmer for 10–15 minutes,
until tender when pierced with a knife. Drain well and return to the pan.
3. Add the miso, ginger, and lemon zest and mash with a potato masher
until smooth. Transfer to a small bowl, cover, and place in the fridge
until ready to use.

LIMA BEAN SPREAD

MAKES ABOUT ½ CUP
KEEPS FOR TWO DAYS IN THE FRIDGE
16-ounce can lima beans, drained and rinsed
2 garlic cloves, peeled and crushed
2 tsp olive oil
1 handful fresh parsley leaves
Juice of 1 lemon

1. Place all the ingredients in a food processor and blend until smooth.
2. Transfer to a bowl, cover, and chill until ready to use.

SWEET CARROT BUTTER

MAKES ABOUT ½ CUP
KEEPS FOR TWO DAYS IN THE FRIDGE OR ONE MONTH IN THE FREEZER
1 pound carrots, trimmed, peeled, and sliced
1 tbsp tahini
2 tsp arrowroot mixed with 1 tbsp cold water

1. Place the carrots in a medium saucepan and cover with water. Bring to a boil, then lower the heat and simmer for 10–15 minutes, until tender when pierced with a knife. Drain well.
2. Blend the carrots in a food processor or with a handheld blender and return to the saucepan.
3. Add the tahini and arrowroot and cook for 1–2 minutes, until thick.
4. Transfer to a bowl, cover, and chill until ready to use.

CASHEW BUTTER

MAKES ABOUT ½ CUP
KEEPS FOR THREE DAYS IN THE FRIDGE
2 cups cashews, soaked in water ovenight
1 tsp tamari sauce

1. Drain the cashews and then place in a food processor with
the tamari and 2 tablespoons of water. Blend until smooth;
you may need to scrape down the sides during the processing.
2. Transfer to a small bowl, cover and place in the fridge
until ready to use.

ALMOND PÂTÉ

MAKES ABOUT ½ CUP
KEEPS FOR THREE DAYS IN THE FRIDGE
2 cups whole almonds, soaked in water overnight
½ cup pine nuts
2 tbsp lemon juice
2 tbsp olive oil
1 clove garlic, peeled and crushed
3 tbsp chopped fresh basil

1. Drain the almonds and place in a food processor with all
the other ingredients and 2 tablespoons of water. Blend until smooth;
you may need to scrape down the sides during the processing.
2. Transfer to a small bowl, cover, and place in the fridge until ready to use.

ASPARAGUS SPREAD

MAKES ABOUT ⅓ CUP

1 bunch asparagus trimmings (tips reserved for a salad)
1 handful fresh herbs such as cilantro or chervil
1 small onion, peeled and roughly chopped
2 tsp miso paste

1. Steam the asparagus for 3–4 minutes.
2. Place all the ingredients in a food processor and blend until smooth.
3. Transfer to a bowl and eat on the same day.

PARSNIP SPREAD

MAKES ABOUT ½ CUP
KEEPS FOR ONE DAY IN THE FRIDGE

3 parsnips, trimmed, peeled, and chopped
2 carrots, trimmed, peeled, and chopped
2 tbsp tahini
2 tsp tamari sauce

1. Place the parsnips and carrots in a medium pan and cover with water. Bring to a boil, then lower the heat and simmer for 10–15 minutes, until tender when pierced with a knife. Drain well.
2. Place in a food processor and blend until smooth. Add the other ingredients and process for another 30 seconds.
3. Transfer to a small bowl, cover, and place in the fridge until ready to use.

BLACK OLIVE TAPENADE

MAKES ABOUT ½ CUP
KEEPS FOR FIVE DAYS IN THE FRIDGE
½ cup drained pitted black olives
2 garlic cloves, peeled and crushed
1 tsp lemon juice

1. Process all the ingredients in a food processor until smooth.
2. Transfer to a clean screw-top jar and place in the fridge until ready to use.

GUACAMOLE DIP

MAKES ABOUT ½ CUP
2 large ripe avocados, pitted, peeled, and chopped
2 spring onions, trimmed and chopped
1 garlic clove, peeled and crushed
1 tbsp chopped fresh cilantro
Juice of 2 limes

Place all the ingredients in a food processor and process until smooth. Eat on the same day.

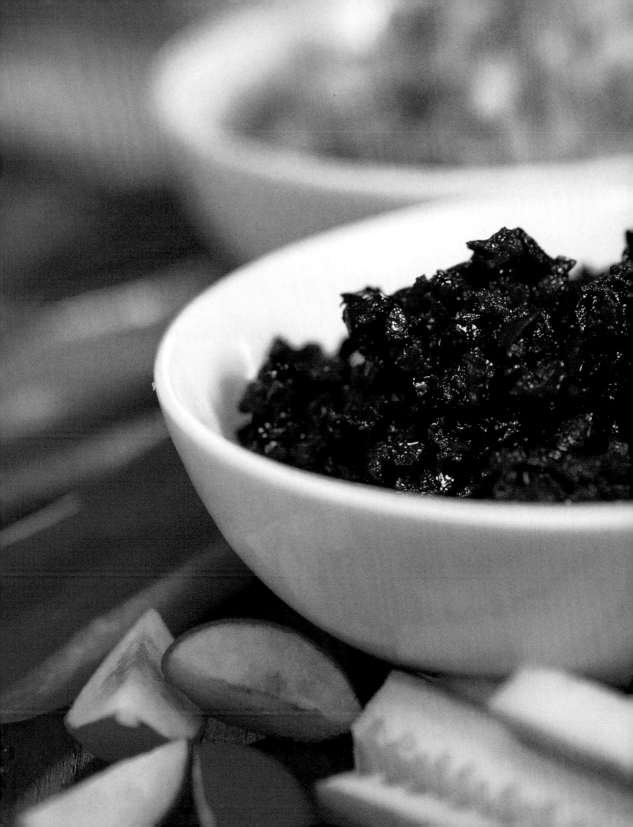

RAW SALSA

MAKES ABOUT ¾ CUP
KEEPS FOR THREE DAYS IN THE FRIDGE
½ pound cherry tomatoes, quartered
4 spring onions, trimmed and finely chopped
1 garlic clove, peeled and chopped
16-ounce can black-eyed peas, drained and rinsed
Juice of 1 lemon
2 tbsp chopped fresh cilantro

Mix all the ingredients together, cover, and chill until ready to use.

TAHINI SALSA

MAKES ABOUT ¾ CUP
2 beefsteak tomatoes, seeded and finely chopped
1 yellow pepper, seeded and finely chopped
1 red onion, peeled and finely chopped
Juice of 1 lime
1 tbsp tahini
2 tbsp sesame seeds

1. Mix the tomatoes, pepper, and onion together in a medium bowl. Add the lime juice and tahini and stir well.
2. Sprinkle with the sesame seeds and eat on the same day.

HOMEMADE HUMMUS

MAKES ABOUT 1 CUP
KEEPS FOR TWO DAYS IN THE FRIDGE
16-ounce can chickpeas, drained and rinsed
1 garlic clove, peeled and crushed
3 tbsp tahini
Juice of half a lemon
2 tbsp chopped fresh cilantro
1 tbsp olive oil

1. Place all the ingredients in a food processor and process until smooth.
2. Transfer to a small bowl, cover, and chill until ready to use.

PICKLE RELISH

MAKES ABOUT ½ CUP
KEEPS FOR FIVE DAYS IN THE FRIDGE
1 onion, peeled and finely chopped
1 green pepper, seeded and diced
1 red pepper, seeded and diced
¼ pound cherry tomatoes, halved
2 tbsp cider vinegar
1 tsp rice syrup

1. Place all the ingredients in a medium saucepan and cook very slowly over gentle heat for 40–45 minutes. Add a little water as needed.
2. Transfer to a clean screw-top jar and allow to cool. Place in the fridge and chill until ready to use.

SWEET POTATO WEDGES

2 sweet potatoes, cut into chunks
1 tbsp olive oil

1. Preheat the oven to 400°F.
2. Bring a large pan of water to a boil, add the sweet potato, and blanch for 4–5 minutes.
3. Drain the sweet potato and return to the pan. Toss well with the olive oil and transfer to a baking sheet.
4. Cook for 25–30 minutes and serve with Guacamole Dip (see page 208) and Raw Salsa (see page 210).

GLUTEN-FREE SQUASH BREAD

1 small butternut squash
2 cups gluten-free flour
2 tsp baking powder

1 tsp herb seasoning (optional)
2 tbsp olive oil

1. Preheat the oven to 400°F.
2. Place the whole butternut squash on a baking sheet and bake for 45 minutes, or until very soft. Cool on the sheet for 30 minutes.
3. Carefully peel the skin from the squash and cut away the stalk. Transfer to a large bowl and break open using a spoon. Scoop out and discard any seeds. Mash well with a potato masher. Measure out ¾ pound and place in a large bowl.
4. Add the flour, baking powder, and seasoning, if using. Stir in ¼ cup cold water and the olive oil and mix together with a large spoon. Place on a lightly floured surface and knead until soft and spongy. Add a little more flour if the mixture is too sticky. Form into a round loaf 6 inches in diameter.
5. Place on a lightly oiled baking sheet and make a cross on the top with a sharp knife. Bake in the oven for 30–35 minutes.
6. Remove from the oven and using oven gloves carefully turn the bread over and tap the base gently. It should sound hollow. If it doesn't, return to the oven and cook for an additional 5 minutes. Serve the bread warm or cold.

MY TOP SNACK FOODS

Here's my list of top snack foods, ranging from fruit and vegetables to sea vegetables and (my all-time favorites) raw nuts and seeds. They're all easily available. Buy organic where possible, and only buy nuts and seeds that are salt- and sugar-free.

► **Dates: The Anti-Stress Snack** These dried fruits are great for helping to relax the body. As with fresh fruit, buy organic where possible.

► **Fruit** This literally means any piece of fresh fruit.

► **Hemp Seeds** Hemp seeds have a smooth nutty flavor and make delicious snacks. The raw shelled ones taste best. Eat them on their own or mixed into avocados, sweet potatoes, or salads. Hemp seeds are an absolutely exceptional source of EFAs and zinc. If you want to feel sexy, then this is the seed for you!

► **Nuts** One of my staple snacks. Try Brazil nuts, the good mood nut, hazelnuts (my favorite), almonds or, in fact, any nut of your choice. You don't need a lot; a few, or a handful, is just right. Nuts are delicious raw, but you can also soak or steam them.
Soaked nuts Soaking raw nuts in water overnight is a good way of enjoying them and makes them easy to digest.
Steamed nuts When you steam nuts (and some seeds too), it gives them a completely different texture and flavor. As an added benefit, nuts that are steamed, as opposed to raw, can be easier to digest. Try steaming cashews or almonds for a completely new taste experience!

► **Pumpkin Seeds** A fantastic source of zinc and EFAs to boost your sex drive. So, don't miss out on them. Try steaming them with soy sauce—fantastic!

► **Sauerkraut** I will let you in on a little secret: my patients love sauerkraut for its ability to increase their sex drive! Try a couple of cupfuls a day to get you started.

► **Soaked Chickpeas** This is one of my favorite snacks. I like to soak them for 24–48 hours and eat them raw in the morning. Leave them for long enough, and they'll start to sprout, maximizing nutrient content and digestibility.

► **Sprouts** Adzuki, alfafa, clover, fenugreek, green pea, lentil, mung bean, quinoa, radish, broccoli seed, sunflower seed, or millet.

► **Sunflower Seeds** My "pick me up" choice in the middle of the day.

► **Toasted Nori Strips** You can buy these from a health food store or bake them in the oven yourself. My kids love to eat these instead of chips. They even take them to school and share them with their friends.

► **Vegetable Sticks or Crudités** Dipped in hummus or one of my delicious spreads. The secret to making veggie sticks appetizing is in the chopping. Don't make the sticks too thick. Nice small, thin sticks are perfect. You can eat lots of them. Cucumbers, carrots, yellow and red peppers, and celery make perfect veggie crudités.

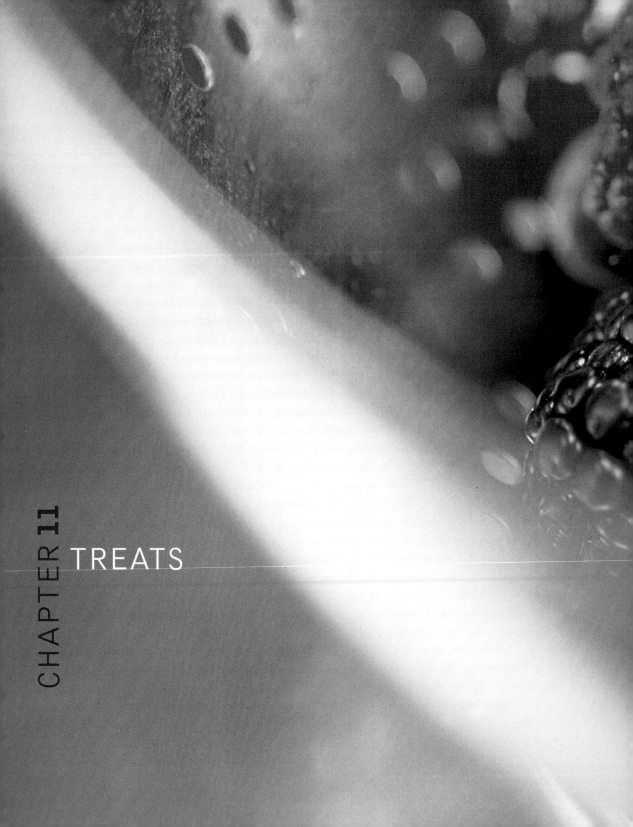

CHAPTER 11

TREATS

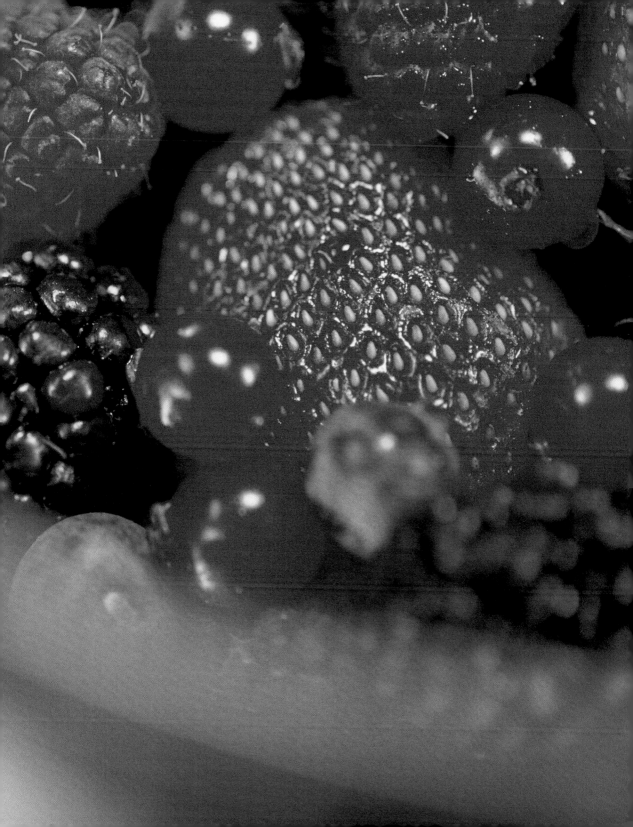

YOU PROBABLY WEREN'T EXPECTING TOO
MANY TREATS, BUT I LOVE TO CREATE HEALTHY
ALTERNATIVES TO SUGAR-LADEN SWEETS AND
PROCESSED FOODS. I DON'T RECOMMEND EATING
THESE TREATS AFTER DINNER, AS THEY ARE
BEST TO DIGEST EARLIER IN THE DAY. SUNDAY
AFTERNOONS ARE MY FAVORITE TIME FOR A
TREAT—THE CAROB FUDGE BROWNIES
(PAGE 225) ARE FANTASTIC!

CHESTNUT CREAM PARFAIT

SERVES 4

4 ounces dried chestnuts, soaked for
12 hours or overnight in cold water
½ cup ground pecan pieces or almonds
1 cup rice milk
2 cups amasake

1 tsp vanilla extract
1 tsp ground cinnamon, plus extra for garnish
¼ tsp ground nut-meg
2 tbsp agar-agar flakes
1 tbsp slivered almonds

1. Put the chestnuts in a medium pan and cover with 1 cup water.
Bring to a boil, then lower the heat and simmer for 20 minutes, or until
tender. Drain and reserve the cooking liquid.

2. Place the chestnuts in a food processor with the pecans or almonds
and process until smooth. Add the rice milk, amasake, vanilla, cinnamon,
and nutmeg and blend until creamy.

3. Heat ½ cup of the reserved cooking liquid and add the agar-agar.
Stir to dissolve and pour into the food processor while it's running.
Blend to combine well.

4. Pour into 4 serving glasses and chill until set. Garnish with slivered
almonds and ground cinnamon.

BLUEBERRY APPLE KANTEN

SERVES 4
1 quart freshly pressed apple juice
6 tbsp agar-agar flakes
1 tsp pure vanilla extract
½ pound fresh blueberries

1. Place the apple juice in a small saucepan and bring to a boil.
Add the agar-agar flakes, then lower the heat and simmer for 2 minutes.
2. Remove from the heat and allow to cool, then add the vanilla.
3. Place the blueberries in a glass bowl, pour over the juice, and chill
for 2 hours in the fridge to set.

LEMON PANNACOTTA

I use the seaweed agar-agar, which makes a clear jelly-like liquid. Because
it tastes neutral, it can be used in both sweet and savory recipes. It is
cooling, so it can help the liver and heat conditions affecting the heart and
lungs.

SERVES 4
2 cups rice milk
Juice and zest of 1 lemon
1 tbsp rice syrup
4 tsp agar-agar flakes

1. Bring the milk, lemon juice, and rice syrup to a boil.
Lower the heat to a simmer and add the agar-agar and lemon zest.
Cook for 3–4 minutes. Remove from the heat and allow to cool.
2. Pour into 4 small molds and chill for 2–3 hours, until set.

CINNAMON RICE PUDDING

This is a fantastic dessert that is loaded with B vitamins. If you are stressed out, need to relax, or just fancy something that is naturally sweet, then this is the best dish going.

SERVES 4
1½ cups long grain brown rice
3 cups rice milk
1 cinnamon stick, broken in half
Juice and zest of 1 lemon

1. Place the rice, rice milk, cinnamon, and lemon juice in a medium pan. Bring to a boil, lower the heat, and simmer for 30–40 minutes, stirring occasionally. Add a little more rice milk if needed. The rice should be very tender and the liquid well absorbed.
2. Serve hot or cold sprinkled with lemon zest.

LEMON MOUSSE

More than half the people who come to see me test low in essential
fatty acids (EFAs)—nutrients you need from your diet. Signs of EFA
deficiency can include dry, rough skin, skin problems, infertility, hair loss,
dry hair, chapped lips, and tiredness. This dessert is a fantastic source of
those much-needed nutrients, mainly because of the avocados, which are
high in EFAs. I often call essential fatty acids essential thinny acids to
induce my clients to eat them. Please banish the fallacy that avocados are
fattening. They are not. They are loaded with good fats, which play a vital
role in weight management. I've combined the avocados here with fresh
dates, which I think of as great anti-stressors. They're yummy too!

SERVES 4
4 whole lemons
4 ripe avocados, pitted, peeled, and mashed
Juice of half a lemon
Juice of half an orange
½ pound pitted dates
2 tbsp maple syrup
Zest of 1 lemon

1. With a very sharp knife, remove the skin from one of the lemons,
leaving the body of the lemon whole. Cut in half and remove the seeds.
Repeat for all the lemons.
2. Place all the ingredients except the lemon zest in a food processor
and process until smooth. Spoon into dessert dishes and chill for 2 hours
in the fridge.
3. Serve garnished with lemon zest.

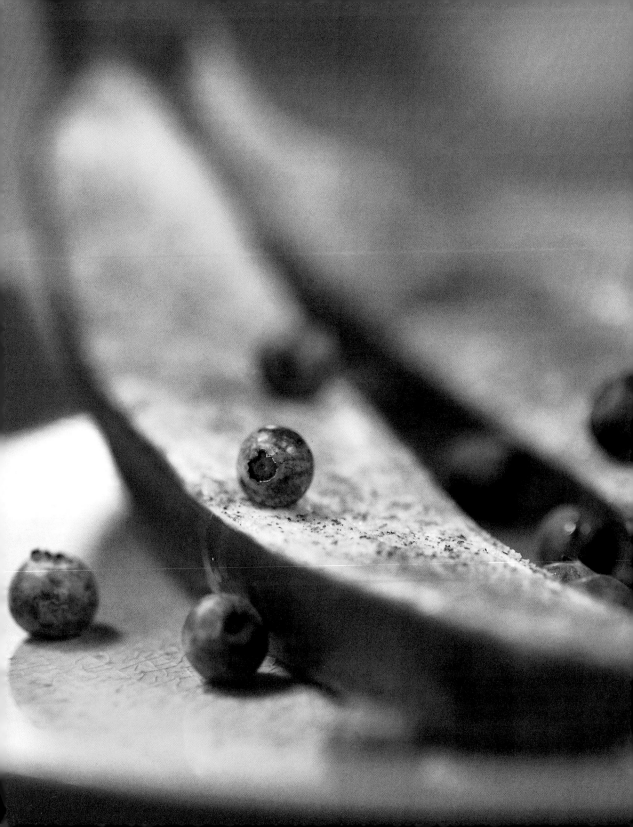

GRILLED BANANA WITH CITRUS SPICE

Researchers have found that three bananas contain enough magnesium to quell a hayfever attack.

SERVES 4
4 bananas, peeled and sliced in half lengthwise
Juice of 1 lemon
2 tsp ground cinnamon
¼ pound fresh blueberries

1. Preheat the oven to 400°F.
2. Place the bananas on a baking sheet, pour over the lemon juice, and sprinkle with the cinnamon.
3. Bake for 10–15 minutes, until caramelized.
4. Serve warm with fresh blueberries sprinkled on top.

These fruit treats are delicious, but remember not to eat fruit as a dessert. For better digestion, enjoy these recipes a couple of hours before/after a meal.

PEARS IN SYRUP

SERVES 4
4 pears, peeled
2 tsp barley malt syrup
2 star anise

1. Place the pears in a pan large enough for them to fit snugly, add the rice syrup and star anise, and cover in boiling water.
2. Bring back to a boil, then lower the heat and simmer for 10 minutes.
3. Allow the pears to cool, then remove them from the syrup.
4. Boil the syrup until it reduces to about ½ cup.
5. Drizzle the thickened syrup over the pears and serve.

BAKED APPLES WITH RAISIN COMPOTE

SERVES 4
4 baking apples, cored and cut in half horizontally
2 tbsp raisins
2 tbsp golden raisins
2 tbsp maple syrup

1. Preheat the oven to 400°F.
2. Place the apples in an ovenproof baking dish.
3. Mix the raisins and golden raisins together and stuff them into the apple cores. Drizzle a little maple syrup into each apple.
4. Bake for 15–20 minutes and serve warm.

LOVERS' PASSION FRUIT DELIGHT

SERVES 4
½ pound fresh strawberries, hulled
4 passion fruit, halved
Fresh mint leaves

1. Slice the strawberries and arrange in a fan shape on a plate.
2. Scoop the passion fruit pulp onto the strawberries, garnish with mint leaves, and serve.

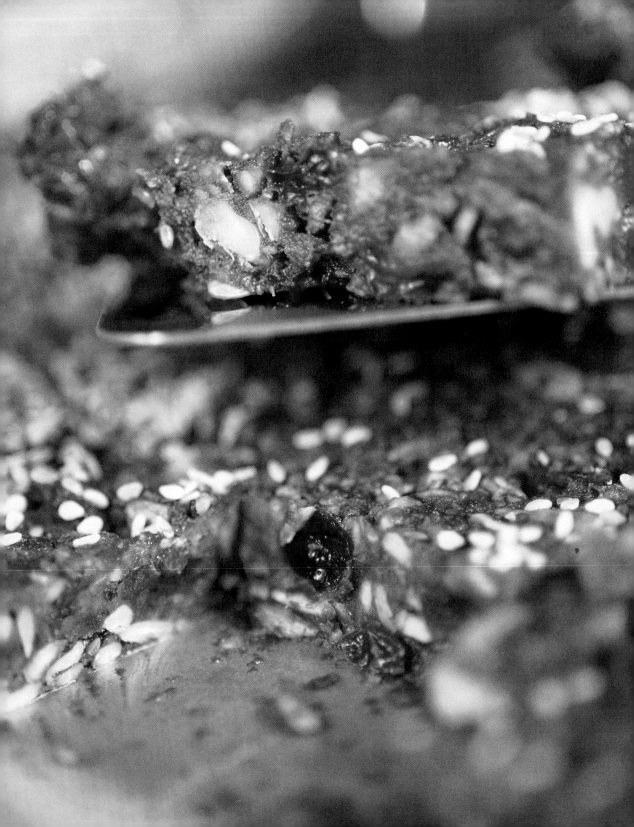

CAROB FUDGE BROWNIES

MAKES 12 PIECES
WILL KEEP IN THE FRIDGE FOR UP TO 5 DAYS
$^3/_4$ **pound pitted dates**
$^1/_2$ **pound soaked raisins**
$^1/_4$ **cup carob powder**
1 pound Brazil nuts, soaked overnight in cold water
$^1/_4$ **pound ground flax seeds**
$^1/_4$ **pound sunflower seeds**
$^1/_4$ **pound chopped walnuts**
$^1/_4$ **pound whole walnuts**
Sprinkle of sesame seeds

1. Place the dates, raisins, carob powder, Brazil nuts, and 2 cups water in a food processor and blend until you have a smooth paste.
2. Mix through the seeds and walnuts.
3. Spread the mixture evenly on to a 5 x 10-inch baking sheet lined with plastic. Sprinkle with sesame seeds, then freeze for 1 hour.
4. Cut into 12 pieces and serve.

CHAPTER 12

STOCKS, SAUCES, AND DRESSINGS

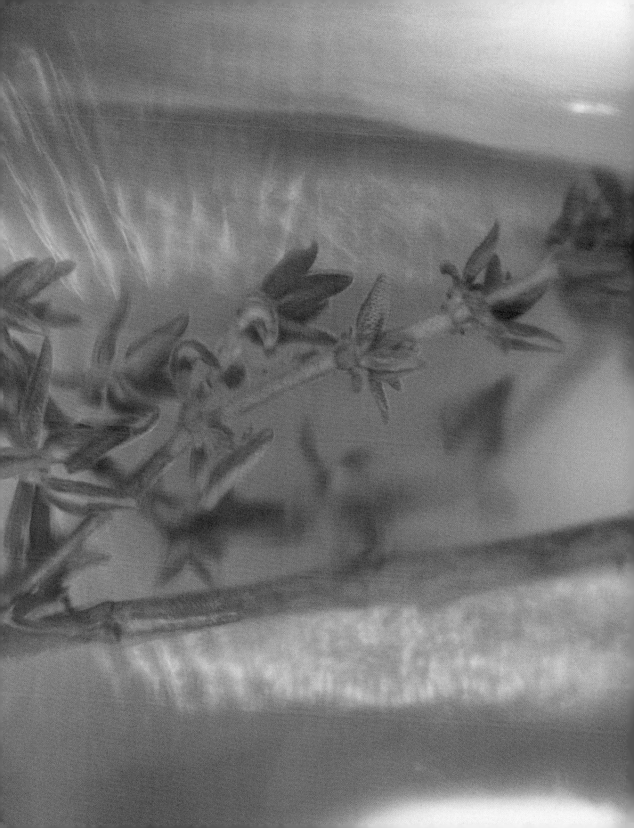

QUICK SALAD DRESSING

Not many people know that ready-made mayonnaise can be thinned down really easily with water to make a simple dressing. This one is flavored with fresh herbs, dill, or mint, for example, but you could use dried herbs or even add finely grated lemon rind for a zesty flavor.

MAKES ¼ CUP
2 tbsp Egg-Free Mayonnaise (see page 233)
2 tbsp chopped fresh herbs

Place the mayonnaise and the herbs in a small screw-top jar along with 2 tablespoons of water, shake well, and serve. This dressing needs to be used on the day of making.

HERBY SALAD DRESSING

MAKES ½ CUP / KEEPS FOR THREE DAYS IN THE FRIDGE

½ cup olive oil	**1 tbsp chopped fresh herbs**
2 tbsp cider vinegar	**¼ tsp wheat-free**
1 tsp Dijon mustard	**vegetable bouillon powder**
Half a garlic clove, peeled and chopped	

Place all the ingredients, together with 2 tablespoons of cold water, in a small screw-top jar and shake well.

SESAME MISO DRESSING

MAKES ½ CUP / KEEPS FOR THREE DAYS IN THE FRIDGE

3 tbsp sesame oil	**1 garlic clove, peeled and crushed**
2 tbsp cider vinegar	**½ tsp chopped fresh basil**
2 tbsp light yellow miso	**½ tsp chopped fresh oregano**

Place all the ingredients, together with 6 tablespoons of cold water, in a small screw-top jar and shake well.

ONION GRAVY

Never underestimate the power of onions. They can aid in the lowering of blood pressure and cholesterol and can keep colds at bay. And my onion gravy makes the Adzuki Bean Stew on page 158 taste out of this world.

MAKES 2 CUPS
KEEPS IN THE FRIDGE FOR THREE DAYS
2 onions, peeled and sliced
1 tsp olive oil
2 tsp tamari sauce
2 tsp arrowroot

1. Place the onions, olive oil, and 6 tablespoons of water in a medium pan and cook gently for 15–20 minutes, until the onions are very soft.
2. Mix the tamari with the arrowroot and add to the onion mixture, along with 2 cups water, mixing well.
3. Cook over medium heat for 10 minutes and serve hot.

VEGETABLE STOCK

MAKES 1 QUART
KEEPS IN THE FRIDGE FOR FIVE DAYS OR IN THE FREEZER FOR A MONTH
1 onion, peeled and sliced
2 leeks, washed, trimmed, and sliced
1 fennel bulb, trimmed, and sliced
2 carrots, trimmed, peeled, and chopped
1 handful fresh parsley stalks
1 tsp coriander seeds
2 fresh bay leaves
2 sprigs fresh thyme

1. Place all the ingredients in a large casserole and pour in boiling water to cover.
2. Bring back to a boil, then lower the heat and simmer for 45 minutes.
3. Strain through a fine sieve and cover. Discard the vegetables.

ROASTED VEGETABLE STOCK

This veggie stock is a great alternative to stock cubes or bouillon powder. Perfect for anyone on a low-salt diet; it's full of rich, natural flavors that will add an amazing zest to your stews and soups. It's also the ideal way to use up a glut of root vegetables, so don't worry if you find yourself throwing in different vegetables each time you make it.

Make this stock in large quantities to save for a later time. Use it as a base for stews and soups. It is already diluted, so there's no need to add any extra water. Just use the same amount of stock as the amount of liquid called for in the recipe.

For easier storage, reduce the stock down to 1 cup and store in ice cube trays in the freezer. Rehydrate 1 cube to 3 parts water.

MAKES 1 QUART
KEEPS FOR ONE WEEK IN THE FRIDGE OR ONE MONTH IN THE FREEZER
6 garlic cloves, unpeeled
3 carrots, trimmed, peeled, and chopped
2 red onions, peeled and quartered
2 parsnips, trimmed, peeled, and sliced
2 celery stalks, trimmed and chopped
1 sweet potato, peeled and chopped
1 leek, washed, trimmed, and thickly sliced
2 sprigs fresh rosemary
1 fresh bay leaf

1. Preheat the oven to 400°F.
2. Place all the ingredients in a roasting pan and roast for 40–45 minutes.
3. Remove the garlic and transfer the other ingredients to a large saucepan. Cover with 1.25 quarts water, bring to a boil, and squeeze the garlic into the stock. Reduce the heat and simmer the stock for 45 minutes.
4. Strain through a sieve and cool.

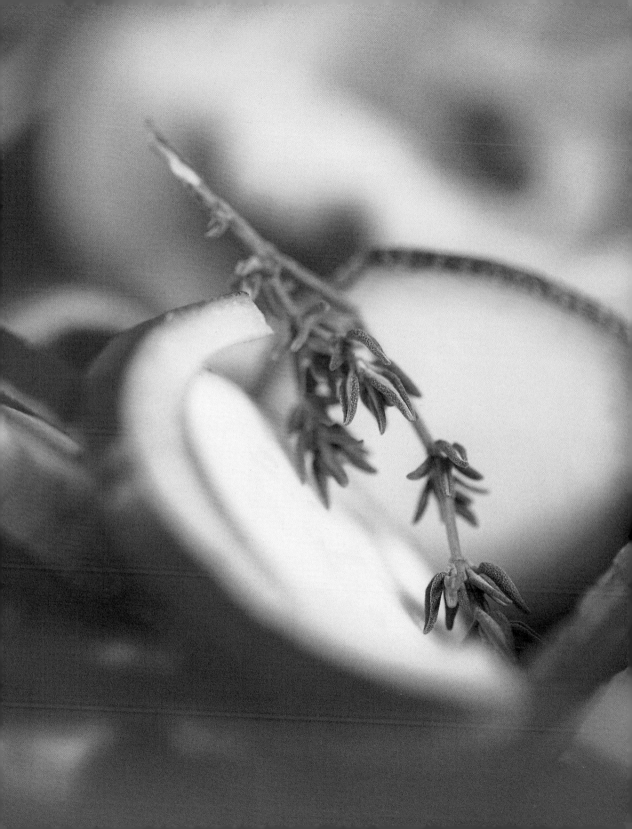

TANGY BARBECUE RELISH

MAKES 1¾ CUPS
KEEPS FOR THREE DAYS IN THE FRIDGE
2 garlic cloves, peeled and finely chopped
1 red onion, peeled and finely sliced
16-ounce can chopped organic tomatoes
1 tbsp chopped fresh basil

Place all the ingredients except the basil in a small saucepan. Bring to a boil, then lower the heat and simmer, stirring occasionally, for 30–40 minutes, until the mixture is soft and syrupy. Add a little water if necessary during the cooking process.

Transfer into a small bowl, cover and chill. Serve with chopped basil.

EGG-FREE MAYONNAISE

MAKES 1½ CUPS / KEEPS FOR TWO DAYS IN THE FRIDGE
⅔ of a 16-ounce block tofu drained, and roughly chopped
1 tbsp olive oil
Juice of half a lemon
1 tbsp cider vinegar (or brown rice vinegar)
1 garlic clove, peeled and crushed

1. Place all the ingredients, together with 2 tablespoons of cold water, in a food processor and blend until smooth.
2. Transfer to a small bowl, cover, and chill.

HOMEMADE KETCHUP

Molasses adds an intriguing sweet flavor and plenty of access to the all-important B vitamins that so many of us are lacking, but you may well find the ketchup sweet enough without it.

MAKES 1¼ CUPS / KEEPS FOR THREE DAYS IN THE FRIDGE
6 ripe tomatoes, quartered
1 red pepper, seeded and chopped
1 small red onion, peeled and chopped
1 garlic clove, peeled and finely chopped
3 tbsp cider vinegar (or brown rice vinegar)
½ tsp molasses

1. Place all the ingredients in a medium saucepan and cook over medium heat for 40 minutes. Stir occasionally and add a little extra water if required.
2. Remove from the heat and cool for a few minutes. Blend in a food processor or with a handheld blender. Pass through a sieve and discard the seeds and pits.
3. Allow to cool, then transfer to a bowl. Cover and chill until ready to use.

FLAVORED OILS

Here are three different flavored oils. Simply fill three sterile bottles with olive oil and add the ingredients by using a wooden skewer to push them under the oil. These oils will keep for one month in a dark cupboard.

ASIAN

2 stalks lemongrass
6 fresh cilantro stalks
1-inch piece fresh ginger

ROSEMARY

1 tsp coriander seeds
3–4 sprigs fresh rosemary

MEDITERRANEAN

2 stalks fresh basil
2 sprigs fresh thyme

2 sprigs fresh oregano
6 garlic cloves, peeled

THE GILLIAN McKEITH FINAL WORD

There's one last secret that you need to know before I sign off. I want you to start thinking about your body as an energy system that absorbs the positive energy of food and our surrounding environment. Many years ago, I used to eat out at a new vegetarian restaurant that opened up in my local neighborhood. The first time I ate there, the food was great and I became a regular. When I went back the following week, I noticed the food tasted downright bad, and on certain days I actually felt a lump in my throat after eating there. Something wasn't right and as it turned out, I learned that the owner was in the kitchen, in a foul mood. She did not want to be there. You could literally tell whether she was there or not from the food.

Conversely, think about the mother who lovingly serves up dinner to her children, or whips up chicken soup when they have a cold. The emotional nourishment and warm healing is immense when the energy is right. So here are your two simple assignments:

First, always prepare your food with a sense of happiness, kindness, compassion, fun, and love. Even if you don't feel so positive before preparing a meal, take a few moments out to shift your mood.

Second, when you go shopping for your fruits and vegetables, take a minute to feel the energy of the produce as well as your own body's energies. Ask yourself, what looks good? What looks healthy? What's screaming out at me? What do I feel like eating today? In this way, you will begin to raise your level of energy consciousness in relation to foods and the body's delicate balance.

Allow this energetic sensitivity to guide your choices of ingredients and how you prepare and serve a meal. This is my greatest discovery for wellness. Until next time ...

Wishing you unconditional Love & Light,

Gillian

XX X

INDEX

239

ACKNOWLEDGMENTS

This cookbook is dedicated to my two dearest wee lassies, who have even gone so far as to sample all of the seaweeds that I advocate and who also put up with my long weekend hours and shifts late into the night writing this book. To Howard, for the most incredible inspiration to share information, for your motivation, words, and help, monumental appreciation and gratitude. Words don't do justice to the enormity of your contribution. By the way, you make the most incredible quinoa porridge.

Much love to Mum and Dad for always believing in me.

ABOUT THE AUTHOR

Gillian McKeith, PhD, is the internationally acclaimed holistic nutritionist and presenter of the hit prime-time television shows *You Are What You Eat* and *Eat Yourself Sexy*. Gillian's television programs are regularly watched by many millions of viewers in more than thirty-five countries around the world. In the United States, Gillian's *You Are What You Eat* TV show airs on BBC America.

With more than four million books now in print, Gillian's *You Are What You Eat* is a runaway bestseller around the globe and has been translated into more than twenty-five languages. Five of her books have gone to number one. She is the author of the American titles *Gillian McKeith's Food Bible*, *Slim for Life*, and *You Are What You Eat*.

Gillian McKeith's mission is to "Empower people to improve their lives through information, food, and lifestyle." Raised in Scotland, Gillian travels extensively giving lectures and seminars to packed audiences. Gillian McKeith, PhD has been working in private practice with clients at the McKeith Clinic in London, England, in the field of food and holistic nutrition for almost two decades.

www.gillianmckeith.com

Gillian conducts wellness and weight-loss retreats in southern Spain.

For more information email retreats@mckeithresearch.com